MENTAL HEALTH

AND

PHYSICAL HEALTH

WHY THEY GO HAND-IN-HAND?

SUSHMITA DUTTA

TRUE SIGN
PUBLISHING HOUSE

Published by True Sign Publishing House
Address: SY. No. 21/2 & 21/3, Sonnenahalli,
Krishnarajapura, Bengaluru,
Karnataka - 560049 India
E-mail: truesignbooks@gmail.com
Website: www.truesign.in

**Mental Health And Physical Health
Why They Go Hand-in-hand?**

Author: Sushmita Dutta

ISBN:978-93-5805-726-3

First Edition: 2023

CONTENTS

Introduction...**5**

1. What is Health? 7

2. What is Mental Health?.. 13

3. Types of Mental Health Disorders 16

4. What is Physical Health?.. 24

5. Benefits of Physical Activity.................................... 26

6. Why is Physical Activity important for Health
   and Well-being?.. 30

7. Connection between Mental and Physical Health 33

8. How your Mental Health affects your Physical Health? 35

9. Importance of Mental and Physical Health............................. 38

10. Youth and the Importance of Physical and Mental Health 41

11. Mental Health In India 46

12. Success Story: A Story of Mental Illness 50

13. Sophie's story – Personal Stories of Depression
    and Anxiety 53

14. Student shares story of Mental Health Struggle
    and Survival 58

15. How does Mental Health affect Physical Health? 62

16. What is Global Health? 65

17. Community Health Problems in India 69

18. How to Solve Major Community Health Problems? 74

19. Health Effects related to Overweight and Obesity 80

20. Global Issues around Physical Activity 84

21. Why we Need to Stop Judging Mental Illness? 88

22. Mental Health in Schools 91

23. If Health is Wealth, Why do we Ignore Mental Health? 94

24. Overcoming the Taboo of Mental Health in India amidst
the Pandemic - Hemant Sethi 99

25. How do Thoughts and Emotions Affect Health? 103

26. Physical Activity Is Good for the Mind and the Body 107

27. Effects of Excess Stress on Physical and Mental Health 111

Conclusion **114**

Introduction

Mental and physical health are two important aspects of our lives. Though they are related, they are different concepts and can affect us in various ways. One problem is that there is a lot of stigma in our society regarding mental healthcare, which can discourage people from seeking professional guidance. It is, therefore, necessary for us to work together to eradicate this stigma and help people better understand how to protect their health.

Difference between Mental and Physical Health

Mental health is just as important as physical health. In fact, our mental health can affect our physical health. For example, if we are not physically active, it can lead to problems such as depression or anxiety. It is important to maintain both our mental and physical health, and to take care of both our body and our mind. Just as there are doctors for treating conditions like heart disease, there are also places that focus on mental healthcare. Many of us are quick to look for help when we have a physical ailment, but fewer people are willing to prioritize caring for their mental health.

Prominent athletes and celebrities like Simone Biles have spoken eloquently about the need for understanding mental health, and people are beginning to listen. If you're experiencing symptoms that are affecting your quality of life, whether they're mental or physical, you owe it to yourself to get evaluated by a qualified medical professional and learn about your treatment options.

Our physical health refers to our physical condition, including our body weight, fitness and health conditions. If you have had a heart condition, you'd want to go and see the best cardiologists in town. Heart problems can be a serious physical issue, but the causes of heart problems can, in some cases, have to do with mental health too. For example, if we are feeling stressed and anxious, that can cause us to have a heart attack or a stroke. Addressing issues like heart problems is important, though we need to learn to respond to our mental health crises with similar urgency.

How can you support your overall health and wellness?

There are some lifestyle changes you can adopt that will protect both your body and your mind. Sleep deprivation can have many negative effects on your health, including increased stress, anxiety, and depression. It can also lead to obesity, heart disease, and diabetes. In addition, sleep deprivation can impair your cognitive function, making it difficult to think clearly and make decisions. If you're struggling to fall asleep , it's a good idea to talk to your healthcare provider to discuss possible solutions.

Therapy is worthwhile even for those who don't have a diagnosed mental health condition. Therapy can help you learn more about yourself, develop new skills, and find relief from stress, anxiety, and other problems. Therapy can be especially helpful if you're going through a difficult time, such as the death of a loved one. It can also help you manage chronic health conditions or deal with other life challenges.

There's a lot to consider when thinking about your health, whether mental or physical. It's also important to understand that mental and physical health may be different, but they aren't completely separate. They can interact, and often mental health conditions can manifest with physical symptoms. If you're experiencing pain, discomfort, or any symptoms that are affecting your daily life or activities, it's always best to get yourself examined by a professional to make sure you don't need any treatment. If you do, then you owe it to yourself to get the care you need, no matter which aspect of your health is of concern.

Chapter - 1

What is Health?

The word 'health' refers to a state of complete emotional, mental and physical well-being. According to the **Centers for Disease Control and Prevention (CDC)**, healthcare costs in the United States were $3.5 trillion in 2017.

However, despite this expenditure, people in the U.S. have a lower life expectancy than people in other developed countries. This is due to a variety of factors, including access to healthcare and lifestyle choices.Good health is central to handling stress and living a longer and more active life.

Types of Health

Mental and physical health are the two most frequently discussed types of health.

Spiritual, emotional, and financial health also contribute to overall health. Medical experts have linked these to lower stress levels and improved mental and physical well-being.

People with better financial health, for example, may worry less about finances and have the means to buy fresh food more regularly. Those with good spiritual health may feel a sense of calm and purpose that fuels good mental health.

Physical Health

A person who has good physical health is likely to have bodily functions and processes working at their peak.This is due not only to absence of disease. Regular exercise, balanced nutrition, and adequate rest - all contribute to good health. People receive medical treatment to maintain the balance, when necessary.

Physical well-being involves pursuing a healthful lifestyle to decrease the risk of disease. Maintaining physical fitness, for example, can protect and develop the endurance of a person's breathing and heart function, muscular strength, flexibility, and body composition.

Looking after physical health and well-being also involves reducing the risk of an injury or health issue, such as:

- minimizing hazards in the workplace

- practicing effective hygiene

- avoiding the use of tobacco, alcohol, or illegal drugs

- taking the recommended vaccines for a specific condition or country when traveling

Good physical health can work in tandem with mental health to improve a person's overall quality of life.

For example, mental illness, such as depression, may increase the risk of drug use disorders. This can go on to adversely affect physical health.

Mental Health

According to the **U.S. Department of Health & Human Services**, mental health refers to a person's emotional, social, and psychological well-being. Mental health is as important as physical health as part of a full, active lifestyle.

It is harder to define mental health than physical health because many psychological diagnoses depend on an individual's perception of their experience.

With improvements in testing, however, doctors are now able to identify some physical signs of some types of mental illness in CT scans and genetic tests.

Good mental health is not only categorized by the absence of depression, anxiety, or another disorder. It also depends on a person's ability to:

- enjoy life
- bounce back after difficult experiences and adapt to adversity
- balance different elements of life, such as family and finances
- feel safe and secure
- achieve their full potential

Physical and mental health have strong connections. For example, if a chronic illness affects a person's ability to complete their regular tasks, it may lead to depression and stress. These feelings could be due to financial problems or mobility issues.

A mental illness, such as depression or anorexia, can affect body weight and overall function.

It is important to approach "health" as a whole, rather than as a series of separate factors. All types of health are linked, and people should aim for overall well-being and balance as the keys to good health.

Factors for Good Health

Good health depends on a wide range of factors.

Genetic factors

A person is born with a variety of genes. In some people, an unusual genetic pattern or change can lead to a less-than-optimum level of health. People may inherit genes from their parents that increase their risk for certain health conditions.

Environmental factors

Environmental factors play a role in health. Sometimes, the environment alone is enough to impact health. Other times, an environmental trigger can cause illness in a person who has an increased genetic risk of a particular disease.

Access to healthcare plays a role, but the WHO suggest that the following factors may have a more significant impact on health than this:

- where a person lives
- the state of the surrounding environment
- genetics
- their income
- their level of education
- employment status

It is possible to categorize these as follows:

- The social and economic environment: This may include the financial status of a family or community, as well as the social culture and quality of relationships.
- The physical environment: This includes which germs exist in an area, as well as pollution levels.
- A person's characteristics and behaviors: A person's genetic makeup and lifestyle choices can affect their overall health.

According to some studies, the higher a person's socio-economic status (SES), the more likely they are to enjoy good health, have a good education, get a well-paid job, and afford good healthcare in times of illness or injury.

They also maintain that people with low socio-economic status are more likely to experience stress due to daily living, such as financial difficulties, marital disruption, and unemployment.

Social factors may also impact on the risk of poor health for people with lower SES, such as marginalization and discrimination.

A low SES often means reduced access to healthcare. A 2018 study in **Frontiers in Pharmacology** indicated that people in developed countries with universal healthcare services have longer life expectancies than those in developed countries without universal healthcare.

Cultural issues can affect health. The traditions and customs of a society and a family's response to them can have a good or bad impact on health.

 Mental Health And Physical Health

According to the **Seven Countries Study,** researchers studied people in select European countries and found that those who ate a healthful diet had a lower 20-year death rate.

The study indicated that people who ate a healthful diet are more likely to consume high levels of fruits, vegetables, and olives than people who regularly consume fast food.

The study also found that people who followed the Mediterranean diet had a lower 10-year all-cause mortality rate. According to the **International Journal of Environmental Research and Public Health,** this diet can help protect a person's heart and reduce the risk of several diseases, including type 2 diabetes, cancer, and diseases that cause the brain and nerves to break down.

How a person manages stress will also affect their health. According to the **National Institute of Mental Health,** people who smoke tobacco, drink alcohol, or take illicit drugs to manage stressful situations are more likely to develop health problems than those who manage stress through a healthful diet, relaxation techniques, and exercise.

Preserving Health

The best way to maintain health is to preserve it through a healthful lifestyle rather than waiting until sickness or infirmity to address health problems. People use the name wellness to describe this continuous state of enhanced well-being.

The WHO defines wellness as follows:"Wellness is the optimal state of health of individuals and groups. There are two focal concerns: the realization of the fullest potential of an individual physically, psychologically, socially, spiritually, and economically, and the fulfillment of one's roles and expectations in the family, community, place of worship, and other settings."

Wellness promotes active awareness of and participating in measures that preserve health, both as an individual and in the community. Maintaining wellness and optimal health is a lifelong, daily commitment.

Steps that can help people attain wellness include:

- eating a balanced, nutritious diet from as many natural sources as possible
- engaging in at least 150 minutesof moderate to high-intensity exercise every week

- screening for diseases that may present a risk

- learning to manage stress effectively

- engaging in activities that provide purpose

- connecting with and caring for other people

- maintaining a positive outlook on life

- defining a value system and putting it into action

The definition of peak health is highly individual, as are the steps a person may take to get there. Every person has different health goals and a variety of ways to achieve them.

It may not be possible to avoid disease altogether. However, a person should do as much as they can to develop resilience and prepare the body and mind to deal with illnesses as they arise.

Chapter - 2

What is Mental Health?

Mental health is all about how people think, feel and behave. Mental health specialists can help people with depression, anxiety, bipolar disorder, addiction and other conditions that affect their thoughts, feelings and behaviors. Mental health can affect daily living, relationships, and physical health.

Stress, depression, and anxiety can all affect mental health and disrupt a person's routine.Although health professionals often use the term mental health, doctors recognize that many psychological disorders have physical roots.

According to the **World Health Organization (WHO)**:"Mental health is a state of mental well-being that enables people to cope with the stresses of life, realize their abilities, learn well and work well, and contribute to their community."

WHO states that mental health is "more than just the absence of mental disorders or disabilities." It is not only about managing active conditions but also looking after ongoing wellness and happiness.It also emphasizes that preserving and restoring mental health is crucial individually and at a community and society level.

In the United States, the **National Alliance on Mental Illness** estimates that almost 1 in 5 adults experience mental health problems each year.In 2020, an estimated 14.2 million adults in the U.S., or about 5.6%, had a serious psychological condition, according to the **National Institute of Mental Health (NIMH).**

Risk Factors for Mental Health Conditions

Everyone is at some risk of developing a mental health disorder, regardless of age, sex, income, or ethnicity. In the U.S. and much of the developed world, mental disorders are one of the leading causes of disability.

Social and financial circumstances, adverse childhood experiences, biological factors, and underlying medical conditions can all shape a person's mental health.Many people with a mental health disorder have more than one condition at a time.

It is important to note that good mental health depends on a delicate balance of factors and that several elements may contribute to developing these disorders.

The following factors can contribute to mental health disruptions.

Continuous social and economic pressure

Having limited financial means can increase the risk of mental health disorders.A 2015 Iranian study describes several socio-economic causes of mental health conditions, including poverty and living on the outskirts of a large city.

The researchers also described **flexible (modifiable)** and **inflexible (non-modifiable)** factors that affect the availability and quality of mental health treatment for certain groups.

Modifiable factors for mental health disorders include:

- Socio-economic conditions, such as whether work is available in the local area
- occupation

      MENTAL HEALTH AND PHYSICAL HEALTH

- a person's level of social involvement
- education
- housing quality
- gender

Non-modifiable factors include:

- gender
- age
- ethnicity
- nationality

The researchers found that being female increased the risk of low mental health status by nearly 4 times. People with a "weak economic status" also scored highest for mental health conditions in this study.

Childhood adversity

Several studies support that adverse childhood experiences such as child abuse, parental loss, parental separation, and parental illness significantly affect a growing child's mental and physical health.

There are also associations between childhood abuse and other adverse events with various psychotic disorders. These experiences also make people vulnerable to post-traumatic stress disorder (PTSD).

Biological factors

The NIMH suggests that genetic family history can increase the likelihoodof mental health conditions as specific genes put a person at higher risk.

However, many other factors contribute to the development of these disorders.Having a gene associated with a mental health disorder does not guarantee that a condition will develop. Likewise, people without related genes or a family history of mental illness can still have mental health issues.

Chronic stress and mental health conditions such as depression and anxiety may develop due to underlying physical health problems, such as cancer, diabetes, and chronic pain.

Chapter – 3

Types of Mental Health Disorders

Some types of mental health disorders are as follows:

- anxiety disorders
- mood disorders
- schizophrenia disorders

Anxiety Disorders

According to the **Anxiety and Depression Association of America,** anxiety disorders are the most common mental illness.People with these conditions have severe fear or anxiety related to certain objects or situations. Most people with an anxiety disorder try to avoid exposure to whatever triggers their anxiety.

Below are some examples of anxiety disorders.

Generalized anxiety disorder

Generalized anxiety disorder (GAD) involves excessive worry or fear that disrupts everyday living.

People may also experience physical symptoms, including:

- restlessness
- fatigue
- poor concentration
- tense muscles
- interrupted sleep

A bout of anxiety symptoms does not necessarily need a specific trigger in people with GAD. They may experience excessive anxiety when encountering everyday situations that do not pose a direct danger, such as chores or appointments. A person with GAD may sometimes feel anxiety with no trigger at all.

Panic Disorder

People with a panic disorder experience regular panic attacks involving sudden, overwhelming terror or a sense of imminent disaster and death.

Phobias

There are different types of phobia:

Simple phobias: These may involve a disproportionate fear of specific objects, scenarios, or animals. A fear of spiders is a typical example.

Social phobia: Sometimes known as social anxiety, this is a fear of being subject to the judgment of others. People with social phobia often restrict their exposure to social environments.

Agoraphobia: This term refers to a fear of situations where getting away may be difficult, such as being in an elevator or a moving train. Many people misunderstand this phobia as the fear of being outside.

Phobias are deeply personal, and doctors do not know every type. There could be thousands of phobias, and what may seem unusual to one person can be a severe problem that dominates daily life for another.

OCD

People with **obsessive-compulsive disorder (OCD)** have obsessions and compulsions. In other words, they experience constant, stressful thoughts and a powerful urge to perform repetitive acts, such as handwashing.

PTSD

PTSD can occur after a person experiences or witnesses an intensely stressful or traumatic event. During this type of event, the person thinks that their life or other people's lives are in danger. They may feel afraid or that they have no control over what is happening.

These sensations of trauma and fear may then contribute to PTSD.

Mood Disorders

People may also refer to mood disorders as affective disorders or depressive disorders.People with these conditions have significant mood changes, generally involving either mania, a period of high energy and joy, or depression.

Examples of mood disorders include:

Major depression: An individual with major depression experiences a constant low mood and loses interest in activities and events that they previously enjoyed (anhedonia). They can feel prolonged periods of sadness or extreme sadness.

Bipolar disorder: A person with bipolar disorder experiences unusual changesin their mood, energy levels, levels of activity, and ability to continue with daily life. Periods of high mood are known as manic phases, while depressive phases bring on low mood. Read more about the different types of bipolar here.

Seasonal affective disorder (SAD): Reduced daylight during the fall, winter, and early spring months triggers this type of major depression. It is most common in countries far from the equator.

Schizophrenia Disorders

The term 'schizophrenia' often refers to a spectrum of disorders characterized by psychotic features and other severe symptoms. These are highly complex conditions.

According to the **NIMH**, signs of schizophrenia typically develop between the ages of 16 and 30. The individual will have thoughts that appear fragmented and may also find it hard to process information.

Schizophrenia has negative and positive symptoms. Positive symptoms include delusions, thought disorders, and hallucinations, while withdrawal, lack of motivation, and a flat or inappropriate mood are examples of negative symptoms.

Early Signs

No physical test or scan reliably indicates whether a person has developed a mental illness. However, people should look out for the following as possible signs of a mental health disorder:

- withdrawing from friends, family, and colleagues
- avoiding activities they would normally enjoy
- sleeping too much or too little
- eating too much or too little
- feeling hopeless
- having consistently low energy
- using mood-altering substances, including alcohol and nicotine, more frequently
- displaying negative emotions
- being confused
- being unable to complete daily tasks, such as getting to work or cooking a meal
- having persistent thoughts or memories that reappear regularly
- thinking of causing physical harm to themselves or others
- hearing voices
- experiencing delusions

Diagnosis

Diagnosing a mental health disorder requires a multi-step process. A doctor may begin by looking at a person's medical history and performing a thorough physical exam to rule out physical conditions or issues that may be causing the symptoms.

No medical tests can diagnose mental disorders. However, doctors may order a series of laboratory tests such as imaging exams and bloodwork to screen for other possible underlying causes.

They will also do a psychological evaluation. This includes asking about a person's symptoms, experiences, and how these have impacted their lives. Sometimes, the doctor may ask a person to fill out mental health questionnaires to get an idea about a person's thoughts, feelings, and behavior patterns.

Most mental health specialists use the **American Psychiatric Association's (APA)Diagnostic and Statistical Manual of Mental Disorders (DSM-5)** to make a diagnosis. This manual contains descriptions and specific criteria to qualify for a diagnosis.

Treatment

There are various methods for managing mental health problems. Treatment is highly individual, and what works for one person may not work for another.

Some strategies or treatments are more successful in combination with others. A person with a chronic mental disorder may choose different options at various stages in their life.

The individual needs to work closely with a doctor who can help them identify their needs and provide suitable treatment.

Below are some treatment options for people with mental ill health.

Psychotherapy or talking therapies

This type of treatment takes a psychological approach to treating mental illness. Cognitive behavioral therapy (CBT), exposure therapy, and dialectical behavior therapy are examples.

Psychiatrists, psychologists, psychotherapists, and some primary care physicians carry out this treatment.

It can help people understand the root of their mental illness and start to work on more healthful thought patterns that support everyday living and reduce the risk of isolation and self-harm.

Medication

Some people take prescribed medications, such as anti-depressants, antipsychotics, and anxiolytic drugs.

Although these cannot cure mental disorders, some medications can improve symptoms and help a person resume social interaction and a routine while working on their mental health.

Some of these medications boost the body's absorption of feel-good chemicals, such as serotonin, from the brain. Other drugs either boost the overall levels of these chemicals or prevent their degradation or destruction.

Self-help

A person coping with mental health difficulties may need to change their lifestyle to facilitate wellness.

Such changes can include reducing alcohol intake, sleeping more, and eating a balanced, nutritious diet. People may need to take time away from work or resolve issues with personal relationships that may be causing damage to their mental health.

People with conditions such as anxiety or depressive disorder may benefit from relaxation techniques, which include deep breathing, meditation, and mindfulness.

Having a support network, whether via self-help groups or close friends and family, can also be essential to recovery from mental illness.

How to maintain your mental health?

Practicing self-care can help improve a person's mental health by reducing a person's risk of illness, increasing energy levels, and managing stress. The NIMH offers several tips to help a person begin with their self-care routine:

Regular exercise: Exercising for 45 minutes, three to five times a week, can significantlyimprove mental health.

Eat a balanced diet and stay hydrated: Eating a nourishing, balanced diet and staying hydrated can give a constant supply of energy throughout the day.

Aim for good-quality sleep: A 2021 review of multiple studies found that more significant improvements in sleep quality led to greater improvements in a person's mental health.

Perform relaxing activities: Breathing exercises, meditation, wellness apps, and journaling can help reduce stress and improve overall health and well-being.

Practice gratefulness: People can practice mindfulness and gratitude by actively identifying things they are grateful for daily.

Challenge negative thoughts: A person can practice positivity by becoming aware of their negative and unhelpful thoughts and challenging them.

Look for positive social interactions: Connecting and maintaining meaningful connections and relationships reduces stress and can also be a source of support and practical help in times of need.

Suicide prevention

If you know someone at immediate risk of self-harm, suicide, or hurting another person:

- Ask the tough question: "Are you considering suicide?"
- Listen to the person without judgment.
- Call the local emergency number, or communicate with a trained crisis counselor.
- Stay with the person until professional help arrives.
- Try to remove any weapons, medications, or other potentially harmful objects.

Outlook

While mental health disorders are common, they vary in severity. Most people can manage their symptoms and lead full lives with the proper treatment and access to support.

For others, recovery may not look like going back to their lives before the mental health disorder but learning new ways to cope and gaining more control over their lives.

The prevalence of mental disorders tends to peak in people ages 18–25, but drops significantly in people aged 50 and over.

Having a mental health problem, especially depression, is strongly associated with severe chronic health conditions such as diabetes, stroke, hypertension, cancer, and heart disease.

The term 'mental health' refers to a person's cognitive, behavioral, and emotional well-being. It affects how people react to stressors, engage with others, and make choices.

According to the **WHO** peak mental health is more than just the absence of mental health problems. It is the ability to manage existing conditions and stressors while maintaining ongoing wellness and happiness.Factors such as stress, depression, and anxiety can all negatively affect mental health and disrupt a person's routine.

Chapter - 4

What is Physical Health?

Physical health can be defined as the normal functioning of the body. It's about how your body grows, feels and moves, how you care for it, and what you put into it.

Pillars of Physical Health

Maintaining good physical health decreases your risk of developing conditions such as heart disease, stroke and some cancers. Being physically healthy also helps you to manage life's challenges by protecting you against fatigue, injury and illness.

Physical health is closely linked to mental health and an integral part of leading a healthy lifestyle and enjoying life. This is often taken for granted and it isn't until we are sick, ill or injured that we put the time and energy in to looking after our physical health. It is important to regularly monitor your overall physical health and getting a check-up if you (or someone you know) are concerned.

The four pillars of health are sleep, nutrition, physical activity and connection.

Sleep

Getting adequate sleep helps to prevent excess weight gain, heart disease and increased illness and disease. Rest and recovery after stressful activity, both mentally and physically, is also important as it enables the body to repair itself and be fit and ready for another day.

Nutrition

Adequate and appropriate nutrition helps support performance, recovery, mental clarity, and overall mood.

Like a vehicle, the body performs best with the right fuel. If you put regular gasoline in a Formula 1 car, it will struggle to compete with the rest of the field and will likely end up making an early pitstop.

Good nutrition provides the body with the nutrients and fuel it needs to perform and recover. It also reduces stress and inflammation in the body, which is associated with injury, illness and mental health issues.

Physical Activity

The body is designed to move. Lack of exercise decreases range of motion within the body's joints causing pain and dysfunction. It also contributes to a decline in physical, mental and physiological health. Sedentary behaviours can lead to a variety of health consequences including weight gain, type two diabetes, cardiovascular disease and mood disorders.

On the other side, too much exercise and stress can have an adverse effect, making the body susceptible to burnout and a compromised immune system. The body functions best with moderate amounts of work, stress and activity, coupled with rest to allow the body to repair and build stronger.

Chapter - 5

Benefits of Physical Activity

Regular physical activity is one of the most important things you can do for your health. Being physically active can improve your brain health, help manage weight, reduce the risk of disease, strengthen bones and muscles, and improve your ability to do everyday activities.

Adults who sit less and do any amount of moderate-to-vigorous physical activity gain some health benefits. Only a few lifestyle choices have as large an impact on your health as physical activity.

Everyone can experience the health benefits of physical activity – age, abilities, ethnicity, shape, or size do not matter.

Immediate Benefits

Some benefits of physical activity on brain health happen right after a session of moderate-to-vigorous physical activity. Benefits include improved thinking or cognition for children 6 to 13 years of age and reduced short-term feelings of anxiety for adults. Regular physical activity can help keep your thinking, learning, and judgment skills sharp as you age. It can also reduce your risk of depression and anxiety and help you sleep better.

Weight Management

Both food eating patterns and physical activity routines play a critical role in weight management. You gain weight when you consume more calories through eating and drinking than the amount of calories you burn, including those burned during physical activity.

To maintain your weight: Work your way up to 150 minutes a week of moderate physical activity, which could include dancing . You could achieve the goal of 150 minutes a week with 30 minutes a day, 5 days a week.

People vary greatly in how much physical activity they need for weight management. You may need to be more active than others to reach or maintain a healthy weight.

To lose weight and keep it off: You will need a high amount of physical activity unless you also adjust your food eating patterns and reduce the amount of calories you're eating and drinking. Staying at a healthy weight requires both regular physical activity and healthy eating.

Reduce your Health Risk

Cardiovascular Disease

Heart disease and stroke are two leading causes of death in the United States. Getting at least 150 minutes a week of moderate physical activity can put you at a lower risk for these diseases. You can reduce your risk even further with more physical activity. Regular physical activity can also lower your blood pressure and improve your cholesterol levels.

Type 2 Diabetes and Metabolic Syndrome

Regular physical activity can reduce your risk of developing type 2 diabetes and metabolic syndrome. Metabolic syndrome is some combination of too much fat around the waist, high blood pressure, low high-density lipoproteins (HDL) cholesterol, high triglycerides, or high blood sugar. People start to see benefits at levels from physical activity even without meeting the recommendations for 150 minutes a week of moderate physical activity. Additional amounts of physical activity seem to lower risk even more.

Some Cancers

Being physically active lowers your risk for developing several common cancers. Adults who participate in greater amounts of physical activity have reduced risks of developing cancers of the:

- Bladder
- Breast
- Colon (proximal and distal)
- Endometrium
- Esophagus (adenocarcinoma)
- Kidney
- Lung
- Stomach (cardia and non-cardia adenocarcinoma)

If you are a cancer survivor, getting regular physical activity not only helps give you a better quality of life, but also improves your physical fitness.

Strengthen your Bones and Muscles

As you age, it's important to protect your bones, joints, and muscles – they support your body and help you move. Keeping bones, joints, and muscles healthy can help ensure that you're able to do your daily activities and be physically active.

Muscle-strengthening activities like lifting weights can help you increase or maintain your muscle mass and strength. This is important for older adults who experience reduced muscle mass and muscle strength with aging. Slowly increasing the amount of weight and number of repetitions you do as part of muscle strengthening activities will give you even more benefits, no matter your age.

Improve your ability to do daily activities and prevent falls

Everyday activities include climbing stairs, grocery shopping, or playing with your grandchildren. Being unable to do everyday activities is called a functional limitation. Physically active middle-aged or older adults have a lower risk of functional limitations than people who are inactive.

For older adults, doing a variety of physical activity improves physical function and decreases the risk of falls or injury from a fall. Include physical activities such as aerobic, muscle strengthening, and balance training. Multi component physical activity can be done at home or in a community setting as part of a structured program.

Hip fracture is a serious health condition that can result from a fall. Breaking a hip have life-changing negative effects, especially if you're an older adult. Physically active people have a lower risk of hip fracture than inactive people.

Increase your chances of living longer

An estimated 110,000 deaths per year could be prevented if adults aged 40 and above increased their moderate-to-vigorous physical activity by a small amount. Even 10 minutes more a day would make a difference.

Taking more steps a day also helps lower the risk of premature death from all causes. For adults younger than 60, the risk of premature death leveled off at about 8,000 to 10,000 steps per day. For adults 60 and older, the risk of premature death leveled off at about 6,000 to 8,000 steps per day.

Manage chronic health conditions & disabilities

Regular physical activity can help people manage existing chronic conditions and disabilities. For example, regular physical activity can:

- Reduce pain and improve function and quality of life for adults with arthritis.
- Help control blood sugar levels and lower risk of heart disease.

Chapter - 6

Why is Physical Activity important for Health and Well-being?

We know that staying active is one of the best ways to keep our bodies healthy. But did you know it can also improve your overall well-being and quality of life?

Here are just a few of the ways physical activity can help you feel better, look better and live better.

It's a natural mood lifter.

Regular physical activity can relieve stress, anxiety, depression and anger. You know that "feel good sensation" you get after doing something physical? Think of it as a happy pill with no side effects! Most people notice they feel better over time as physical activity becomes a regular part of their lives.

It keeps you physically fit and able.

Without regular activity, your body slowly loses its strength, stamina and ability to function properly. It's like the old saying: you don't stop moving from growing old, you grow old from stopping moving. Exercise increases muscle strength, which in turn increases your ability to do other physical activities.

It helps keep the doctor away.

Too much sitting and other sedentary activities can increase your risk of heart disease and stroke. One study showed that adults who watch more than 4 hours of television a day had an 80% higher risk of death from cardiovascular disease.

Being more active can help you:

- lower your blood pressure
- boost your levels of good cholesterol
- improve blood circulation
- keep your weight under control
- prevent bone loss that can lead to osteoporosis

All this can add up to fewer medical expenses and medications later in life!

It can help you live longer.

People who are physically active and have a healthy weight live about seven years longer than those who are not active and are obese. And the important part is that those extra years are generally healthier years! Staying active helps prevent chronic illnesses and diseases associated with aging. So active adults maintain their quality of life and independence longer as they age.

Here are some other benefits you may get with regular physical activity:

- Helps you quit smoking and stay tobacco-free.
- Boosts your energy level so you can get more done.

- Helps you manage stress and tension.

- Promotes a positive attitude and outlook.

- Helps you fall asleep faster and sleep more soundly.

- Improves your self-image and self-confidence.

- Helps youspend more time outdoors.

The **American Heart Association** recommends at least 150 minutes of moderate-intensity aerobic activity each week. You can knock that out in just 30 minutes a day, 5 days a week. And every minute of moderate to vigorous activity counts toward your goal.

Chapter - 7

Connection between Mental and Physical Health

There are multiple connections between mental health and physical conditions that significantly impact people's quality of life, demands on healthcare and generate consequences to society. The **World Health Organization (WHO)** defines: health as a state of complete physical, mental and social well-being and not merely the absence of disease or infirmity. The WHO states that "there is no health without mental health."

Nowhere is the relationship between mental and physical health more evident than in the area of chronic conditions. The associations between mental and physical health are:

- Poor mental health is a risk factor for chronic physical conditions.

- People with serious mental health conditions are at high risk of experiencing chronic physical conditions.

- People with chronic physical conditions are at risk of developing poor mental health.

The social determinants of health impact both chronic physical conditions and mental health. The key aspects of prevention include increasing physical activity, access to nutritious foods, ensuring adequate income and fostering social inclusion and social support. This creates opportunities to enhance protective factors and reduce risk factors related to aspects of mental and physical health.

Understanding the links between mind and body is the first step in developing strategies to reduce the incidence of co-existing conditions and support those already living with mental illnesses and chronic physical conditions.

Chapter - 8

How your Mental Health affects your Physical Health?

The link between mental health and physical health is often misunderstood. They're often thought of as separate entities, but the two go hand in hand. In fact, the **World Health Organization** defines health as a state of complete physical, mental and social well-being.

The perceived disconnect between "mind" and "body" creates the misconception that mental illness is not a physical disease. In reality, mental health has a direct impact on your physical health.

Many of us are not aware of how common mental illness is. About one in five adults has a mental illness in any given year. Mental illness is more than just being depressed. It covers a wide range of problems, spanning from ones that affect mood to those that affect thinking or behavior. Examples include:

- Depression
- Anxiety disorders
- Schizophrenia
- Eating disorders
- Bipolar depression
- Addictive behaviors

Connecting the Mind and Body

You might be wondering how does my mental health affect my physical health? Well, poor mental health can affect your ability to make healthy decisions and fight off chronic diseases.

What's more, neglecting your mental health can lead to more serious health complications such as:

- Heart disease
- High blood pressure
- Weakened immune system
- Asthma
- Obesity
- Gastronomical problems
- Premature death

Depression alone can cause chronic fatigue, insomnia and increased sensitivity to aches and pains due to abnormal function of neurotransmitters in the brain.

Tips to create a healthy body and mind

Just taking care of your mind isn't the best way to improve your mental health. Here are some ways you can improve your mental and physical health:

Exercise regularly.

Exercise can ease depression and anxiety. Choose a form of exercise that works for you. This may be a mindful and intention-driven yoga practice .

Eat a healthy diet.

Diets loaded with processed foods have been linked with increased depression and anxiety. Avoid skipping meals, which can lead to fatigue and unhealthy snacking. Try to include fruits, vegetables, nuts, whole grains, fish and healthy fats, like avocados, into your meals. This will be helpful for increased brain function.

Maintain a normal sleep schedule.

Not getting enough sleep has been linked with depression, anxiety and stress. Adults require seven or more hours of sleep per night. If you're having trouble falling and staying asleep, try one of the following:

- relaxing before bed

- lowering your caffeine intake, or

- setting a stricter schedule for bedtime

- Get support.

Your social circle is also a vital aspect to preventing a decline in mental health. But mental health can be a difficult topic to discuss with peers. This often prevents people from seeking help. Don't be afraid to reach out to friends and family for support.

Don't Wait to Get Help

In many cases, people seek out a mental health expert only after a crisis has occurred. According to a 2016 study by the **Columbia University Medical Center**, less than a third of American adults who screened positive for depression received treatment for their symptoms. Getting help earlier can prevent mental health conditions, like depression and anxiety, from developing.

If you are experiencing symptoms of any mental health condition, it is important to contact a medical professional who can help you. Eating right and exercising can help some people improve their mental health. However, others may need medication or counseling to see changes. By partnering with a medical expert, you will be better able to find out what's right for you.

Chapter - 9

Importance of Mental and Physical Health

Mental health is important for overall well-being. The things that we do physically also impact us mentally, and it's important to be aware of both physical and mental health. In this way, you can achieve overall well-being. The connection between physical health and mental health is more than what you think it is. Taking good care of your physical health is proven to have a positive impact on your mental health and well-being. On the other hand, however, if your mental health declines, then your physical health might decline as well.

Why is physical and mental health important?

Having good physical health helps lessen the symptoms of depression; while on the other hand mental health disorders can lead to worse physical health. The intrinsic relationship between physical health and mental health means that staying physically fit and healthy is important. However, some people struggle to maintain good health, for example, the elderly, in healthcare and community service settings.

Living a sedentary lifestyle may also cause serious illnesses such as cancer, even though it can be treated in therapy centres.

Having a healthy lifestyle can help prevent the worsening of mental health conditions such as depression and anxiety. Heart disease, diabetes, obesity, and other chronic health problems can also be prevented by having a healthy lifestyle. Stress management, getting enough sleep, staying fit and active, and eating healthy food are important factors to improve your overall physical and mental health.

The relationship between physical and mental health

We can always distinguish and differentiate the 'body' from the 'mind'. But when it comes to physical health and mental health, there is a strong relationship between the two.

Having poor physical health can lead to a higher risk of developing mental health problems, and having poor mental health can negatively impact our physical health, which leads to a higher risk of chronic conditions.

Lifestyle factors

Stress. Everyone experiences stress in their lives, but no one likes to be stressed out because of the effects that it can have. Stress is a normal part of our lives. We experience stress when we're doing things too much or we don't get enough rest. We also experience stress when we worry about certain things like money, relationships, a friend, or a loved one going through difficult circumstances or struggling with an illness. Knowing how to manage stress can be a change for you, with a positive impact on your physical and mental health. Meditating and reflecting is a good start for managing stress.

Sleep. Your physical, mental, and emotional health depend on how well you rested. Sleep is essential for having good physical and mental health. It also plays a role in our moods, ability to learn, organ health, in our immune system, and other body functions such as metabolism and hormone release.

Diet. The food you intake can have an impact on your overall physical and mental health. Eating nutritious food can have a positive effect on your way towards a healthy lifestyle. Also, emotions like anger, sadness, or joy, your brain can react to signals from your stomach which makes that gut-wrenching feeling at the pit of your stomach. This is also a reason to eat a nutritious and balanced diet so that your stomach and brain can be healthy, and function properly.

Exercise. Doing physical activity in any form is a good way to keep you physically fit and healthy, and as well as improve your mental health. Research shows that doing physical activity influences the release of the happy hormone called endorphins. Even gentle forms of exercise such as brisk walking can increase mental alertness, energy, positive mood, and it can significantly improve your quality of life.

Benefits and the impact of being physically fit on your mental health

Being physically active is not just about increasing aerobic capacity and muscle size, it can improve your physique, trim your waistline, and improve your physical health. That is not the reason why people keep motivated to do physical activity. People exercise because it gives them a sense of well-being, being energetic throughout the day, and medicine for challenging mental health problems.

Exercising regularly can have an extremely positive impact on depression, anxiety, and ADHD. Even the most basic exercise can benefit you big time. No matter the age or fitness level, exercising can be a powerful tool to deal with mental health problems, and improve your overall sense of well-being.

Even the elderly can do minimal exercises while using their medical equipment to prevent injuries. Exercising can also sharpen your memory and thinking, boost your self-esteem, get you a good night's sleep, a boost of energy, and you can have a stronger resilience in your life.

Chapter - 10

Youth and the Importance of Physical and Mental Health

The most important portion of any nation's workforce is its youth. It is believed that investing in education, wellness, and rights could lead to tremendous socio-economic development with a large youth population. No wonder today's youth will be innovators, creators, builders, and leaders of tomorrow.

There are approximately 1.8 billion adolescents and young people between the ages of 10 and 24 in the world today. Investing in their health and education can change their lives and positively impact their economy and society. India is now one of the world's most young countries, with over 62 percent of its working-age (15–59 years) and over 54 percent of its total people below twenty-five. The average age of the Indian population is expected to be 20 in 2020, compared to 40 in the US, 46 in Europe, and 47 in Japan. This population advantage gives an advantage over other nations when we speak of demographic dividends. Today's youth are becoming increasingly restless, working hard to close the gaps.

Youngsters Health and Nutrition

Following are the main health problems that adolescents face:

Injuries and wounds

Adolescents are very much susceptible to unintentional injuries. Accidents have accounted for countless lives in the previous years. Unfortunately, many of them were just innocent pedestrians and cyclists. As a way forward, we as responsible citizens need adherence to road safety laws that strengthen road laws.

Violence

Interpersonal violence accounts for nearly one-third of all adolescent male deaths in low- and middle-income countries globally. Interpersonal brutality is among the most significant cause of death among the youth worldwide. Its importance varies significantly by region of the world.

Mental well-being

There are many determinants to juvenile well-being and mental health. Violence, exclusion, living in sub-humanitarian and fragile settings can add to one's probability of developing mental health problems. Failure to address these would mean an invite to mental health consequences that last into adulthood, affecting physical and psychological health and restricting opportunities to live fulfilling lives as grown-ups.

Nutritional deficiencies

Iron deficiency affects youth, especially female youth. Iron and folic acid supplementation is a viable solution that promotes health before adolescents become parents. Besides, regular hygiene is the need of the hour that prevents micro-nutrient deficiencies.

Healthy eating habits formed in adolescence lay the groundwork for good health in adulthood. Reduced marketing of foods high in saturated fats, trans fats, free sugars, or salt and increased access to healthy foods is vital for everyone, especially for children and adolescents.

Obesity and malnutrition

Many boys and girls in developing countries enter adolescence malnourished, putting them at risk of disease and premature death. On the otherhand, the proportion of adolescents who are overweight or obese is growing in the middle and high-income countries. Diarrhea, lower respiratory tract infections (pneumonia), and meningitis are the top three causes of adolescent mortality.

Physical exercise

Adolescents benefit greatly from physical activity in various aspects such as cardio-respiratory health, muscular fitness, bone health, maintaining healthy body weight, and psycho-social & mental health. The **World Health Organization** recommends that adolescents should engage in at least 60 minutes of moderate- to vigorous-intensity physical activity per day, including play, games, sports, and exercise (such as cycling or walking) or physical education.

Calories in a Balanced Diet

Human beings require different amounts of calories to be active and maintain a healthy weight. The number of calories you need depends on whether you are male or female, your genes, age, height & weight, whether you are still growing, and how active you are, which may vary from day-to-day.

Controlling how much and what types of food you eat and the beverages you consume is part of healthy eating. Youth must supplement their diet with fruits, vegetables, fat-free or low-fat dairy foods, whole grains, low-fat protein foods against choices that are high in sugar, salt, and unhealthy fats.

Fruits and Vegetables

Dark green, red, and orange vegetables are high in nutrients like vitamin C, calcium and fiber. Adding tomato and spinach or any other available greens to your sandwich is a simple way to increase the number of vegetables in your meal.

Grains

Instead of refined grains, white bread, and white rice, choose whole grains such as whole-wheat bread, brown rice, oatmeal, and whole-grain cereal.

Protein

Increase your protein intake by eating low-fat or lean meats like turkey or chicken, as well as other protein-rich foods like seafood, egg whites, beans, nuts, and tofu.

Dairy

Build strong bones by drinking low-fat milk. If you can't digest lactose opt for lactose-free milk or calcium-fortified soy milk. Youth can try taking low-fat or fat-free yogurt as an integral of their balanced diet.

Fats

Fat is an essential component of your diet. Fat aids in the **growth and** development of your body, the health of your skin and hair. However, fats have more calories per gram than protein or carbohydrates, and some are unhealthy. Some fats, such as plant oils liquid at room temperature, are better than others. Avocados, olives, nuts, seeds, and seafood such as salmon and tuna fish are high in healthy oils.

Say 'No' to Sugar Substitutes

Fruit is naturally sweet. Other foods, such as ice cream and baked desserts, and some beverages, contain added sugars to enhance their sweetness. These sugars contribute calories but no vitamins or fiber. Consume no more than 10% of your daily calories from added sugars in food and beverages. Instead of a candy bar, choose an apple or a banana.

Get Enough Rest

It can be challenging to get enough sleep, especially if you have a job, or are involved in other activities after school. Getting enough sleep, like eating healthy and getting enough physical activity, is essential for staying healthy. To perform well in school, work and drive safely, and fight infection, you must get enough sleep. You may become moody and irritable if you do not get enough sleep. Research has found that a lack of sleep may contribute to weight gain.

Caring for your Health

The role of youth in nation-building is critical. They are problem solvers who make a positive difference in the lives of other young people and the nation, and they are highly ambitious. They can forge their own identity while also propelling the country forward. However, they will be unable to do so without the assistance of the family, community, government, and other young people.

Chapter - 11

Mental Health In India

Mental health is about a person's mental and emotional well-being. Being mentally sound would mean that one possesses a balanced mind, confidence and self-esteem. A mental illness is a problem that significantly affects how a person thinks, perceives and reacts.

There are different kinds of mental illnesses that vary in degrees and severity. It can be divided into **common mental illnesses** and **severe mental illnesses**. Mental health illness can range from psychosis– which is a chemical imbalance in the body to neurosis– which is poor attitudinal learning during the growing or formative years.

Common Mental Health Illnesses include:

- Depression

   MENTAL HEALTH AND PHYSICAL HEALTH

- Anxiety/Phobias

- Eating Disorders

- Stress

Severe Mental Health Illnesses Include:

- Schizophrenia

- Bipolar disorder

- Clinical depression

- Suicidal tendency

- Personality disorder

Statistics show that 1 in every 5 individuals suffers from some form of mental health illness symptoms. 50% of mental health conditions begin by age 14 and 75% of mental health conditions develop by age 24. Mental illness can be triggered by multiple factors. Complex interactions between mind, body and environment result in psychological disorders. Some of the factors are long term acute stress, biological factors, drug abuse and overdose, cognitive behaviour like constant negative thoughts, low energy, etc, social problems like financial problems, breakdowns, isolation, etc.

Symptoms of mental health illness are:

- Persistent negative thoughts including a preoccupation with death or suicide

- Difficulty concentrating

- Low energy or severely fluctuating energy levels

- Hearing voices

- Wanting to spend excessive amounts of time alone

- Inappropriate and uncontrollable behaviour: excessive anger or sadness, for example

- Severe paranoia

Mental health in India is still a fairly new topic and the mental health myths and taboos attached to this subject are prevalent to this date. According to the **National Health Programme** by the **Ministry of Health and Family Welfare**, 6% of Kerala's population has mental disorders. 1 in a 5 has some emotional and behavioural problems. Close to 60 to 70 million people in the country suffer from common and severe mental disorders. India is the world's suicide capital with over 2.6 lakh cases of suicide in a year. WHO statistics say the average suicide rate in India is 10.9 for every lakh people.

There are a few reasons:

Ignorance: The first and foremost reason being awareness and knowledge. People use words like 'mad' and 'asylum' carelessly. There are far too many derogatory and demeaning terms used to describe someone who is mentally not fit and this stigma coupled with ignorance and lack of awareness discourages people who are suffering to speak up and reach out for help.

Lack of help: We have just 43 state-run mental health institutions across the country. 3800 psychiatrists available as against the requirement of 11,500; 898 clinical psychologists as against 17250, 850 psychiatric social workers as against 23000, 1500 psychiatric nurses as against 3000. That means there is only one psychiatrist for four lakh Indians and only 1,022 college seats for mental health professionals are set aside in India.

No insurance for the mentally ill: Insurance companies do not provide medical insurance to people who are admitted to hospitals with mental illnesses. Admission to a good hospital is out of reach for some because of this. A good treatment doesn't come cheap and without insurance cover, it becomes even more difficult.

How the pandemic has aggravated conditions?

India's statistics related to addressing mental health issues were poor, always. It was made worse by the COVID-19 pandemic as the first wave spread across the world in 2020. How did it happen?

- Long periods of isolation
- Frontline workers not being able to come physically close to their family members
- Loss of job
- Financial difficulty
- Not being able to see or meet loved ones
- Alcohol and substance abuse due to stress
- Fear of the unknown
- Cloud of uncertainty

- Constantly worrying about getting infected and infecting people around you
- Not being able to express oneself
- Having to work overtime, complete disruption of work-life balance
- Losing loved ones due to the infection
- Increase in domestic violence
- Closed institutions

All these points mentioned above heightened the critical situation of unaddressed mental health already existing in India. Although the pandemic presented a great opportunity in the form of work from culture to spend time with one's family and loved ones (who earlier had to deal with periods of separation due to pressing work commitments), not all people received the same benefit or felt the same about having to work from home.

The negative impact of the pandemic felt by the greater portion of the country became prominent in the form of anxiety, depression, burnout and a tendency to commit suicide. Many young people in India who had taken loans at the time of the pandemic from unregulated sources were unable to meet these loans and out of embarrassment and constant humiliation were pushed to the brink of suicide.

Significant efforts were taken by the government to raise awareness and address issues earlier pushed aside due to fear of associated stigma. Many programmss such as the **National Mental Health Program, District Mental Health Program** and mental health institutions such as the **National Institute of Mental Health and Neuro-Sciences** and **Central Insitute of Psychiatry** encouraged people to reach out and seek assistance with the help of the national helpline number in times of need.

Needless to say that the pandemic has been hard on everyone as it exposed gaps in our lives and presented many new unforeseen challenges.

Mental illness can be treated with the right kind of support, for psychosis illnesses, the right medication under the right guidance is very important and for neurosis illness, getting good counselling, support and love from peer circle and family plays a crucial role. Reaching out or identifying these problems at an early stage is very important.

Chapter – 12

Success Story: A Story of Mental Illness

The onset of the disease was insidious, but even today, I still vividly remember the painful episode in my life. I completed high school, college, and medical school with great success. Everything seemed set, and I was about to start a residency program at a prestigious institution. It seemed as if my hard work had paid off and my dreams were realized. However, six weeks into my residency, I was in trouble. I was repeatedly unable to complete my work in a timely fashion. In fact, I did almost everything, including walking down the hall and going to the bathroom, at a very slow pace. In addition, I had trouble concentrating on even the simplest of tasks. Having always been blessed with an excellent memory, I noted with dismay that I was often unable to recall basic facts I had read. It was a frustrating time, since it had always been very important to me to do my work in a conscientious manner. Despite the demoralizing effect the ensuing negative feedback had on me, I resolved to overcome the hurdle. It was a very frustrating struggle, because no matter how hard I tried, I could not improve. I remained slow, inefficient, disorganized, and was almost always late — very late. It seemed as if my mind was paralyzed and I was condemned to play the role of the worst resident in the program. Slowly I began to wonder if I was contracting some sort of dementia.

Eventually I decided to schedule a medical workup to rule out any disease that could possibly be causing my symptoms. I desperately almost hoped that I would be vindicated by the diagnosis of some physical ailment. Instead, I was diagnosed with depression. Curiously, the diagnosis did not come as much of a relief. My condition proved to be a very isolating experience, and the isolation only intensified the disease and its accompanying shame and loneliness. I knew that many people — even some in the health profession — regarded depression as a character flaw rather than a true illness. Depression would not exculpate me for my dismal performance as a resident in the same way, for example, a brain tumor would. Depression would not relieve me of the guilt about having failed at my job in the same way a diagnosis of hypothyroidism would. Most importantly, I could not talk to my peers about the pain of depression as I could if I suffered from migraine headaches or a bleeding stomach ulcer. However, the diagnosis did allow me to finally receive proper treatment with medication and psychotherapy. It was at this time that I found out about Physician Health Services (PHS) in Massachusetts.

My participation in the weekly meetings at PHS as well as my sessions with my counselor played a very important role in my road to recovery. For the first time in my life, I was surrounded by people who understood what it was like to go through life with depression. Though I am shy by nature, I was able to share my experiences with fellow physicians and find comfort and empathy instead of judgment. In turn, their inspiring stories gave me hope and strength, and I began forming friendships. The kind, helpful, and understanding individuals at PHS gave me the chance to see myself as a person with depression rather than a worthless resident, and allowed me to trade in the sentiment of shame for a sense of accomplishment and pride in battling the pain of depression. The PHS contract was another valuable element of my professional rehabilitation, because it provided me with a structured program through which I could formally document my recovery under the guidance of my PHS associate director and designated monitors at work. The contract validated my illness, and I considered the successful completion of the contract a major milestone in my recovery.

It was at about this time, two years after my initial diagnosis of depression, that I was diagnosed with colon cancer. While cancer provided me with another very unexpected hurdle in life, I also got the chance to experience, in juxtaposition, society's starkly different reactions to mental and physical disease. The same individuals who regarded my depression somewhat skeptically reacted with shock and ensuing full-hearted support in response to my cancer diagnosis, and I never had to explain to anyone that I was in pain. I finally had a reason to be sad. Interestingly enough, so far, my depression brought me far worse pain and suffering than the colon cancer has, yet, unlike the latter, the former leaves no visible scars on the body for others to see. The wonderful people at PHS provided me with a lot of help and support, promoting my recovery at no cost to me. To the many health professionals who face illnesses that leave them impaired at work, organizations such as PHS represent one of the few avenues in our society through which they can achieve recovery and themselves promote the healing of others.

Success Story: A Personal Story of Mental Illness

Massachusetts Medical Society

https://www.massmed.org › Physician_Health_Services

Chapter – 13

Sophie's story – Personal Stories of Depression and Anxiety

Hello, my name is Sophie and I am a mother of two. I want to share with you my personal story of recovery. Just keep in mind that this is my story and that it's not my intention to say that this is how it should be done. Everyone is different, everyone's personal circumstances are unique and we all have to find our own path to getting better. You can only draw from other people's experiences.

I have had depression before so I was already aware that my general practitioner (GP) could help me in some way. It was also my choice to see him because I felt that I needed to talk to someone who knew what depression was and because I felt that I needed medication.

My GP was very thorough in his assessment and careful to prescribe me the right medication. When I was pregnant he consulted with a psychiatrist before prescribing my medication. At first I went to see him 3 times a week so he could monitor how I was, and with each visit he gave me adequate time to voice my concerns.

He also referred me to a psychologist urgently when I had my first episode of antenatal depression (I had it during both pregnancies). Over the years I have built up a very good relationship with my GP and I still see him from time to time to touch base and discuss the issues surrounding my depression. I still take medication and need to have a review from time to time.

Seeing a psychologist

My first visit to a psychologist was shortly after I was diagnosed with antenatal depression. It was scary to start with because I felt so overwhelmed with negative feelings. I kept going every week though and soon felt that it was one of the best things I could have done for myself.

I so badly needed to talk to someone about all the weird things I was feeling and thinking. I really needed his support and to hear that I was "normal". I also learned that I had many issues to deal with such as childhood and family issues. It became clear that it was really important for me to do therapy for those issues in order to help myself get better.

Looking back, I often wonder how I made it to 30 without any therapy. I truly felt like an emotional cripple when I had my first major episode of depression. In therapy I gained an enormous amount of self-awareness. I feel like I know myself properly now and by gaining that renewed identity, I have learned new ways of coping with the issues in my life.

Confiding in other people

That was a hard one. Of course, my husband knew I wasn't well, but I found it hard to tell him how unwell I really was. I was ashamed of the fact that I couldn't cope and blamed it on myself. After learning more from the psychologist and later psychiatrist, I realised that I'm not to blame and I started to tell my husband more and more how I felt.

That was hard to do, and has caused a lot of emotional upheaval between us at times, but it was necessary. The more I opened up, the more he understood and the more supportive he became. I may make it sound easy, but it actually took years to achieve. We still struggle at times with the fact that we don't understand each other's needs but when we take the time and effort to express to each other how we feel, we always seem to work it out.

I was very lucky that I had some very good friends whom I could confide in when I started feeling depressed. I will be forever thankful for their support and kindness. I have to say that even though I have wonderful friends, it is great to be able to talk to people who have experienced depression as well. Feeling depressed is such a hard thing to explain to someone. People with similar experience just 'know' and that makes me feel 'normal' and accepted.

What I got out of confiding in other people is the knowledge that no matter how I feel I will still be accepted for who I am. That was so powerful. It allowed me to be me, dark clouds and all. I didn't get that response from everyone though. Some people simply didn't understand. That was okay too as long as they weren't negative towards me.

To clean or not to clean...

I hate housework. It seems a never-ending chore that I can never get on top of. I used to be so tidy and neat but now I have had to adjust my standards dramatically to cope with 2 kids.

It has taken me years but I finally came to the conclusion that it's okay to have a messy house. I stressed about that a lot. Constant housework only makes me grumpy and I resent the fact that I don't get to have time for anything enjoyable. Slowly over the years, I have managed to get my priorities right (and what feels good for me). My house is never super clean and tidy, but at least I manage to have some time for myself every day. I clean it when it suits me or when it really needs to be done and that makes me feel good too. Nobody else seems to mind what my house looks like either.

What do I really like to do?

By the time my second child was about 5 months, I felt yet again stuck at home. I figured that the best way to get some quality "me" time was to go out somewhere for a few hours to a place where they had a crèche. I enrolled in a mosaics course at a local community centre with a crèche. I had a fantastic time and so did the kids. I love being creative and it relaxes me enormously. It helps me get out of a negative frame of mind sometimes and gives me great pleasure.

Yoga

I decided to give yoga a go because a friend of mine had told me it was very good for your overall health – physical and emotional. I didn't hold out much hope though because I am the stiffest most inflexible person I know. I absolutely loved it. Gaining more flexibility came but that was only a minor benefit. I realised that yoga had given me a sense of control over myself. The exercises require you to find a balance and become aware of your body, which was quite an eye-opener. I wasn't so bad at it after all. Each session finished with half an hour meditation which seemed to recharge my energy and at the same time, was peaceful. Yoga made me feel a lot stronger and more able to deal with negativity.

Maintenance

It has been just over 6 years since I was first diagnosed with antenatal depression. I can now say that I've almost recovered, but not totally. The experience of depression has truly changed my entire life. I had to take a long, hard and painful look at myself including how I was neglecting to look after myself.

I compare feeling depressed with the feelings of a 5-year-old who didn't know how to look after herself in this big bad world. I was so incredibly scared and just wanted someone to take me by the hand and cuddle and hold me until I felt better. The bad news was that people could only nurture me for short periods of time such as like the 1 hour sessions with a psychologist instead of for a whole month. I just had to learn how to do it for myself.

It was so incredibly hard and I felt like giving up many times. I don't even know how I got through some of the really bad days, but somehow I did. I reached a point where I became determined not to be beaten by this damn illness; I deserved happiness and my family deserved a happy wife and mother.

So very slowly the clouds started to lift and my mood became better for slightly longer periods of time. I still had days when any effort of gaining enjoyment out of life seemed hopeless, but they became less frequent. I had to pull all my strength together to find ways of improving my life and that meant changing. Changing everything it seemed … from the way I perceived myself to changing the way I cleaned my house. I needed to find a balance between looking after myself and looking after my family. I had to come to terms with the fact that I am by no means perfect. I have flaws like every other human being on this planet and that is perfectly okay!

By maintenance I mean that I have to constantly remind myself of what is important in my life, what makes me happy and how to set my priorities accordingly. Maintenance requires ongoing effort but is nowhere near as hard as recovering from depression. For example, I am still taking antidepressant medication. When I reduced my medication about a year ago I felt depressed within a period of two months. Together with my GP we decided it was better to take the full dosage of medication because it enables me to lead a normal life. The bottom line is at least I have now learned to do whatever it takes to be healthy. I have gained happiness and feel that my life is very worthwhile and wonderful.

Chapter - 14

Student shares story of Mental Health Struggle and Survival

As I was driving home down the back roads of the-middle-of-nowhere, Oklahoma, my tears and screams could only momentarily be interrupted by the pills I was washing down with whatever water had been left in my car. It took everything in me to not swerve off the road, thinking about how mad my parents would be if I wrecked the car. Those intrusive thoughts of "I could just flip this car" snuck into my mind nearly every time I drove a car.

The 20-minute drive home felt like hours of pure pain that I couldn't wait to escape, but when I got home, I wasn't moving. I just wasn't getting out of my car. After another numbing half-hour of stillness, I finally got out of the car and started aggressively pacing around the street. My mother came outside, and, between anguished cries, I begged her to take me to the hospital.

Now, this wasn't just one psychotic break. I hadn't been living my life as the pretty cheerleader, student councilor-turned-sorority girl I appeared to be. So much more lay under my skin.

My battle with mental health began before I can truly remember. There are tales out there of early elementary school teachers bringing up concerns of anxiety to my parents because I showed major signs. Looking back, I agree.

I hated the thought of change and could not cope with it in the slightest. Whenever I had a substitute teacher, I would complain of a stomachache; when my church got a new priest, I was petrified; when I found out my dad interviewed for a job in Washington and we could soon be moving, I was traumatized. All these things, big or small, caused me to lie awake at night and let the anxiety course through my veins.

Although those feelings started so early, the real trouble didn't start until middle school, when the bullying set in. As an outgoing and positive child, I strived to live my life with a constant smile. The world didn't agree.

Even though the comments and abuse went over my head at the time, they still hurt. The degrading comments from my family and constant feeling of living in my older sister's shadow added to the hurt. The daily smile I put on my face was real, but so was the pain. Each battle was one I could win, but when the names started becoming vulgar and the threats started becoming violent and the inappropriate passes started to become physical, I started to become weak and I started to lose.

High school came with more battles but better hiding places. When I first got to school in the mornings, I would immediately go straight to my favorite teacher's classroom and sit in the corner on the floor. At the time I had some made-up reason as to why I was doing so, but it was really because I was hiding from all the hurt. Occasionally, I'd find a small group of friends, but they were some of the most toxic and harmful to me. After a week with who I thought loved and supported me, I'd retreat back to my home base of a classroom.

I got very involved in high school. My best friend likes to say I was the Rachel Berry of our high school because I was super talented and involved, but everyone hated me for no reason. I didn't watch Glee so I didn't understand that reference, but people who did think it's fitting. Although I cheered and was on the student council, my real passions were in the orchestra and Youth and Government.

The list of involvement goes on and on with track and field, poetry club, student political groups, dance, theater and Girl Scouts and on and on. I seldom had an ounce of freedom and I loved it. Less free time meant less time to think about the pain I felt.

With high school graduation came time to say goodbye to all my old organizations and the old me. I was ready to start anew. I confidently walked across the stage with the most genuine smile I had produced in a long time and I felt a sigh of relief. My days of agony were over, right? The summer after my senior year would only bring me joy. My days were filled with (joyous) freedom, smiles and art. I worked at a children's theater camp where I met someone, and for the next year he would be my heart and soul.

Jumping into my freshman year at Oklahoma State was hard to say the least. I was eager to go through the Greek recruitment process, but it did not go how I hoped. As my week carried on and my number of houses stayed very high, I was surprised to get a knock on my door one morning from one of my recruitment councilors telling me I had been released from every single house. A wave of horror hit me that I still occasionally feel to this day where I am reminded that out of 13 sorority houses, not a single one wanted me. That was a painful pill to swallow. Now don't get me wrong, I am thankful for how things ended up working out because I did decide to go through the Continuous Open Bidding process and I now belong to a wonderful sisterhood that I absolutely love. But there are some feelings you just can't shake.

Once college really got into full swing the story gets a little complicated. I spent nearly every weekend in Oklahoma City with my boyfriend who I thought was helping me but was slowly diminishing my mental health little by little. I had very few friends until November when I met a small group of people from an organization I was involved with who are still some of my closest friends, yet I kept shoving them to the side because my priorities were with my boyfriend. Lastly, I was studying something I hated. Coming into college, I had this very clear idea of what I wanted to do, but I very quickly realized it was not at all what was going to make me happy. However, I was terrified to change my major because that concept of change had petrified me so often before.

The culmination of these challenges led me to my breaking point. With the pressure building and building, I couldn't help but crack and crumble until one day I completely gave up and gave in.

But I do want to say there is hope. After my attempt, I spent a week in a mental hospital, and I came out on the other side alive. I came out breathing with a heartbeat and the ability to love and hug and smile and kiss and dance and remind people how beautiful they are. I came out on the other side. That is irreplaceable.

Talking to someone helps. Whether it's a friend, a parent, a professor or a licensed professional, it helps and it is so worth it. Taking prescribed medication has helped me as well. Taking medication can be really scary and it may be difficult to find the correct dosage and combination for you, but it is so worth it once you do. My path to finding the right medicine for me was not as challenging as it may be for some because I regularly met with the psychiatrist at University Health Services on campus. Although I was nervous to go at first, the ease and vastness of the treatment and care on campus was astounding to me. Oklahoma State truly cares about its students and I see it every single day in my professors, my employers, my advisors and my peers.

The first thing you try may not be right, but the first pair of shoes you try on may not be right either. You'll still find the right chunky white sneakers, so don't give up.

It's OK to say "no." It's OK to take a day for yourself. It's OK to not be OK. If there's one thing I've learned through all of this, it's that you are loved, I promise you that. And even if you feel like the entire world hates you right now, I still love you.

Student shares story of mental health struggle and survival

Oklahoma State University

https://news.okstate.edu › articles › communications

Chapter - 15

How does Mental Health affect Physical Health?

Although the mind and body are often viewed as being separate, mental and physical health are actually closely related. Good mental health can positively affect your physical health. In return, poor mental health can negatively affect your physical health.

Effects of Mental Health on Physical Health

Your mental health plays a big role in your general well-being. Being in a good mental state can keep you healthy and help prevent serious health conditions. A study found that positive psychological well-being can reduce the risks of heart attacks and strokes. On the other hand, poor mental health can lead to poor physical health or harmful behaviors.

Chronic diseases. Depression has been linked to many chronic illnesses. These illnesses include diabetes, asthma, cancer, cardiovascular disease, and arthritis. Schizophrenia has also been linked to a higher risk of heart and respiratory diseases.

Mental health conditions can also make dealing with a chronic illness more difficult. The mortality rate from cancer and heart disease is higher among people with depression or other mental health conditions.

Sleep problems. People with mental health conditions are more likely to suffer from sleep disorders, like insomnia. Insomnia can make it hard to fall asleep or stay asleep. Insomnia leads to breathing problems, which can cause you to wake up frequently.

Around 50% to 80% of people with mental health conditions will also have sleeping problems. Only 10% to 18% of the general population experience sleeping problems.

While conditions like depression, anxiety, or bipolar disorder may lead to sleep problems, sleep problems can also make existing mental health conditions worse.

Smoking. People with mental health conditions are more likely to smoke than those who do not have mental health conditions. Among smokers, people with mental health conditions are more likely to smoke a greater number of cigarettes.

People with depression have lower levels of the chemical dopamine. Dopamine influences positive feelings in your brain. The nicotine in cigarettes triggers the production of the chemical dopamine, so smoking may be used as a way to relieve symptoms of depression.

However, since nicotine only offers temporary relief, you may feel a recurring need to smoke, which may lead to possible addiction.

Access to healthcare. People with mental health conditions are less likely to have access to adequate health care. It may also be more difficult for people with mental health conditions to take care of their physical health When you have a mental health condition, it can be hard to seek care, take prescriptions regularly, or get enough exercise.

Physical Health conditions that may affect Mental Health

Your physical well-being also has an impact on your mental health. People with physical health conditions may also develop mental health conditions.

Psoriasis is a dermatological condition characterized by painful red sores on the skin. It is associated with acute stress and depression.

Individuals with psoriasis experience emotional and psychological distress that negatively impacts their overall health and quality of life. Stress and depression mainly come from anxiety, stigma, and rejection.

Being diagnosed with cancer or having a heart attack can also lead to feelings of depression or anxiety. Around one-third of people with serious medical conditions will have symptoms of depression, such as low mood, sleep problems, and a loss of interest in activities.

How to take care of your Mental and Physical Health?

If you want to improve your general well-being, you should take care of both your physical and mental health.

Here are some ways to take care of yourself physically and mentally:

Get regular exercise. Exercise is important for keeping physically fit, but it can also help improve your mood. A daily 10-minute walk may increase your mental alertness leaving you energetic and in a good mood.

Eat a proper diet. A diet high in fruits and vegetables and low in processed sugars or fats can make you feel better physically and mentally. Avoid alcohol and drugs. Although drinking and smoking may make you feel better in the short term, they can have a negative effect on both your physical and mental health.

Get enough sleep. A good night's sleep is around seven to nine hours for adults. You can also take a 30-minute nap during the day to feel more alert.

Try relaxation techniques. Meditation, deep breathing, and focusing your thoughts can all help when you are feeling stressed.

Develop good mental practices. Try to focus on positive emotions and events rather than negative ones.

Seek help from others. Talking with friends or family members can help you feel less stressed. Getting others to help with difficult situations can also reduce the burden you feel.

Chapter – 16

What is Global Health?

The effects of a globalized economy, advances in transportation, and changes to agricultural practices have resulted in health care issues transcending international borders.

The first step to understanding global health is to define it, and then learn about some related issues. It includes the study, research, and practice of medicine with a focus on improving health and health care equity for populations worldwide.

While the **World Health Organization (WHO)** is one of the most prominent agencies advancing global health, researchers and leaders in a variety of fields are spearheading initiatives to work together.

Prominent global health issues to be aware of

1. Pandemics

According to the **World Health Organization**, pandemics are defined as global disease outbreaks. Examples of pandemics include certain influenza outbreaks, COVID-19, and other viral threats that reflect our vulnerability to widespread diseases—many of which originate in animals.

Every year, there are newly emerging pandemic threats. Vaccination efforts can help, but it's critical to address issues at the source by addressing important areas like health education and responsible agricultural practices. Researchers have also made recommendations on global risk mitigation measures that can help even after an outbreak occurs.

2. Environmental factors

How can air pollution and climate change affect the health of the human population? In most cases, the answer lies in water sources and sanitation.

Storms, flooding, droughts, and air pollution make it easier for diseases to spread across large groups of people. The immediate solution is to provide resources like bottled water and sanitation technology, but global health must also focus on the prevention of environmental challenges in the first place.

"Climate change is thought by many global health experts to be the greatest threat to human health," Dr. Macpherson says. "Global policies to mitigate mankind's contribution to climate change are gaining traction."

"Such changes will have profound health benefits for those who live in urban centers, which account for more than 50 percent of the world's population," Macpherson explains.

3. Economic disparities and access to healthcare

Despite relentless progress in the field of medicine, communities across the world still lack access to basic health education and health care. This results in health disparities, such as high infant mortality rates, which are often related to geography. Other disparities are the result of income inequality, with individuals and families simply unable to afford health care that is otherwise unavailable.

To solve these economic challenges, global health professionals must explore opportunities to uplift underrepresented communities in public health forums, encourage physicians to practice in remote areas, and introduce policies that reduce barriers and increase access to health care.

4. Political factors

As conflicts within or between nations destroy critical infrastructure, average citizens become more vulnerable to diseases. This leads them to seek opportunities to flee the dangerous situations that threaten their well-beings.

Migration can allow illnesses to quickly spread, but organizations like the WHO stress that solutions should aim to improve refugee and migrant health through efforts like organizing across borders to endorse policies that bridge short-term humanitarian crisis responses with long-term health care access improvements.

5. Non-communicable diseases

Heart disease, stroke, cancer, diabetes, and other non0communicable diseases (NCDs) account for 70 percent of all deaths worldwide, according to the WHO.

Education plays a role in the prevention of NCDs, helping populations understand and change lifestyle factors, such as poor diets, inactivity, tobacco use, and alcohol consumption. But there is also a correlation between income level and the prevalence of NCDs.

The WHO notes that 85 percent of premature NCD-related deaths occur in low- and middle-income countries. Reducing the number of NCDs globally means reducing the factors that disproportionately arise in lower-income communities.

6. Animal health, food sourcing, and supply

Agricultural practices, including irrigation, pesticide use, and waste management, can influence animal health, making disease transmission a concern at every stage of the food supply chain. With pathogens originating from animals or animal products playing such a significant role in disease transmission, veterinary medicine must be included in any effort to improve global health.

Opportunities to influence global health

The ever-growing list of global health issues can be overwhelming, but there are so many ways individuals can make a positive impact.

"Everyone can make a difference," Dr. Macpherson asserts. "Small contributions quickly add up if enough people take up the cause."

One suggestion is to expand your perspective on medicine by attending global health speaking events or pursuing an international education, particularly if you are a practicing MD or a prospective medical student. SGU, for instance, empowers students to pursue opportunities in global health by offering a dual MD/MPH degree. This option allows them to gain perspective on integrating medical care at both the holistic and patient levels.

Chapter - 17

Community Health Problems in India

Major Health issues:

India is one of the pioneers in health service planning with a focus on primary healthcare. In 1946, the Health Survey and Development Committee, headed by Sir Joseph Bhose recommended establishment of a well structured and comprehensive health service with a sound primary health care infrastructure. Social development through improvement in health status can be achieved through improving the access to and utilization of Health, Family Welfare and Nutrition service with special focus on underserved and under privileged segment of population.

Under the Constitution, health is a state subject. Central Government can intervene to assist the state governments in the area of control/eradication of major communicable and non-communicable diseases, broad policy formulation, medical and Para-medical education combined with regulatory measures, drug control and prevention of food adulteration, Child Survival and Safe Motherhood (CSSM) and immunization programme.

However, there are numerous health problems in India, like water supply and sanitation continue to be a challenge, only one of the three Indians has access to improved sanitation facilities such as toilet. India's HIV/AIDS epidemic is growing threat. Cholera epidemics are not unknown. The maternal mortality in India is the second highest in the world. India is one of the four countries worldwide where polio has not yet been successfully eradicated and one third of the world's tuberculosis cases are in India. Three out of four children who died from measles in 2008 were in India. According to the World Health Organization 900,000 Indians die each year from drinking contaminated water and breathing in polluted air. Following are some of the major community health problems in India.

Malnutrition:

According to a 2005 report, 42% of India's children below the age of three were malnourished, which was greater than the statistics of sub-Saharan African region of 28%. Although India's economy grew 50% from 2001–2006, its child-malnutrition rate only dropped 1%, lagging behind countries of similar growth rate. Malnutrition impedes the social and cognitive development of a child, reducing his educational attainment and income as an adult. These irreversible damages result in lower productivity. Major nutritional problems in India are Protein Energy Malnutrition (PEM), Iodine Deficiency Disorder (IDD), Vitamin-A deficiency and anemia.

High infant mortality rate:

Approximately 1.72 million children die each year before turning one. The under five mortality and infant mortality rates have been declining, from 202 and 190 deaths per thousand live births respectively in 1970 to 64 and 50 deaths per thousand live births in 2009. However, this decline is slowing. Reduced funding for immunization leaves only 43.5% of the young fully immunized. A study conducted by the **Future Health Systems Consortium** in Murshidabad, West Bengal indicates that barriers to immunization coverage are adverse geographic location, absent or inadequately trained health workers and low perceived need for immunization. Infrastructure like hospitals, roads, water and sanitation are lacking in rural areas. Shortages of healthcare providers, poor intra-partum and newborn care, diarrheal diseases and acute respiratory infections also contribute to the high infant mortality rate.

Diseases:

Diseases such as dengue fever, hepatitis, tuberculosis, malaria and pneumonia continue to plague India due to increased resistance to drugs. In 2011, India developed a totally drug-resistant form of tuberculosis. India is ranked 3rd highest among countries with the amount of HIV-infected patients. Diarrheal diseases are the primary causes of early childhood mortality. These diseases can be attributed to poor sanitation and inadequate safe drinking water in India. India also has the world's highest incidence of Rabies.

However in 2012 India was polio-free for the first time in its history. This was achieved because of the Pulse Polio Programme started in 1995-96 by the government of India. Indians are also at particularly high risk for atherosclerosis and coronary artery disease. This may be attributed to a genetic predisposition to metabolic syndrome and adverse changes in coronary artery vasodilatation. NGOs such as the Indian Heart Association and the Med win Foundation have been created to raise awareness of this public health issue.

Poor sanitation:

As more than 122 million households have no toilets, and 33% lack access to latrines, over 50% of the population (638 million) defecate in the open.(2008 estimate.). This is relatively higher than Bangladesh and Brazil (7%) and China (4%). Although 211 million people gained access to improved sanitation from 1990–2008, only 31% use the facilities provided. Only 11% of Indian rural families dispose of stools safely whereas 80% of the population leave their stools in the open or throw them in the garbage. Open air defecation leads to the spread of disease and malnutrition through parasitic and bacterial infections.

Safe drinking water:

Access to protected sources of drinking water has improved from 68% of the population in 1990 to 88% in 2008. However, only 26% of the slum population has access to safe drinking water, and 25% of the total population has drinking water on their premises. This problem is exacerbated by falling levels of groundwater caused mainly by increasing extraction for irrigation. Insufficient maintenance of the environment around water sources, groundwater pollution, excessive arsenic and fluoride in drinking water pose a major threat to India's health.

Kala Azar:

Kala-azar is a serious public health problem. Kala-azar control was being provided by the Government of India out of the **National Malaria Eradication Programme (NMEP),** until 1990-91. The Centre provides insecticide, anti-Kala-azar drugs and technical guidance to the affected states.

Female health issues:

Women's health in India involves numerous issues. Some of them include the following:

Malnutrition: Most Indian women are malnourished. The average female life expectancy today in India is low compared to many countries. In many families, especially rural ones, the girls and women face nutritional discrimination within the family, and are anemic and malnourished. The main cause of female malnutrition in India is the tradition requiring women to eat last, even during pregnancy and when they are lactating.

Breast cancer: One of the most severe and increasing problems among women in India, resulting in higher mortality rates.

Stroke: Polycystic ovarian disease (PCOD): PCOD increases the infertility rate in females. This condition causes many small cysts to form in the ovaries, which can negatively affect a woman's ability to conceive.

Maternal mortality: the maternal mortality in India is the second highest in the world. Only 42% of births in the country are supervised by health professionals. Most women deliver with help from women in the family who often lack the skills and resources to save the mother's life if it is in danger. According to UNDP Human Development Report, 88% of pregnant women (15-49) were found to be suffering from anemia.

Rural health : Rural India contains over 68% of India's total population, and half of all residents of rural areas live below the poverty line, struggling for better and easy access to health care and services. Health issues confronted by rural people are many and diverse – from severe malaria to uncontrolled diabetes, from a badly infected wound to cancer. Postpartum maternal illness is a serious problem in resource-poor settings and contributes to maternal mortality, particularly in rural India.

Chapter – 18

How to Solve Major Community Health Problems?

Major Community Health Problems

1. Pollution

Pollution is one of the major concerns of the country. It has consistently posed a lot of threat to environment as well as hazards to human health and welfare. This is manifested by the prevalence of diseases and the quality of environment incurred by irresponsible citizens.

The pollution problem should not be shouldered by a sole agency directly controlling it. The **Department of Environment and Natural Resources** should be assisted by other government agencies, local government units and government organizations to create and set-up guidelines in its control and management. Dissemination of information will also be an instrument in helping implement such strategies contributory to the solution of the problem.

2. Improper disposal of human excreta and sewage

Improper disposal of human excreta and sewage has been responsible for many epidemics on record which have brought sickness and death to a large number of people. It is also one of the most important factors responsible for the high incidence of gastro-intestinal infections including intestinal paratism in a community.

3. Improper refuse storage and disposal

The improper storage and disposal of waste material or refuse is also responsible for the spread of communicable diseases and production of insects such as flies, rats, mosquitoes, etc. It will also create foul odor in the community.

4. Food sanitation

Food sanitation deals largely with health hazards and the sanitary features of food handling. It also concerns with the quality and protection of food values, and with technological and even economic aspects of the food handling processes to fully accomplish its aim of disease prevention.

5. Control of rodents and insects

The control of rodents, insects and related household pests, commonly called vectors, have public health significance for they are also cause of spread of communicable diseases. It is important to minimize their number and/or eliminate them from household premises.

Proper ways of Storage, Garbage Disposal, Recycling

Refuse is solid and semi-solid waste materials other than human excreta. Waste material in refuse may be divided into:

a. Garbage - left-over vegetable, animal and fish material from kitchen and food establishments. These materials have a tendency to decay giving off foul odors. They also serve as food for flies and rats.

b. Rubbish - waste material such as bottles, broken glasses, tin cans, waste papers, discarded porcelain wares, pieces of metal, and other wrapping materials.

c. Ashes - left over from burning of wood and coal. Ashes may become a nuisance because of the dust associated with them.

d. Dead animals - dead dogs, cats, rats, pigs, chickens usually run over by vehicles on streets and public highways. They also include small and other large animals that died from diseases.

e. Stable manure - animal manure from stables.

f. Street sweeping - dust, manure, leaves, cigarette butts, waste papers, and other materials that are swept from streets.

g. Night soil - human waste normally wrapped and thrown into sidewalks and streets.

h. Yard cuttings - leaves, branches, grass, and other similar materials produced during cleaning of gardens and also after storms.

The amount of refuse produced is affected by many factors such as climate, season of the year, industries present, economic condition of the family, and geographical location.

The satisfactory handling of refuse may be considered under three headings, namely: storage, collection, and disposal.

House Storage

The proper storage of waste material is very important if we are to prevent flies, rats, and other insects from being attracted to these wastes and prevent foul odors.

Proper storage of waste materials especially garbage will require containers that are:

a. Small enough to be easily carried when filled with waste.

b. Sufficient in number to store all the waste materials produced between collection times

c. Provided with tight-fitting covers so that flies and rats cannot get in and so that fouls odors in the home and community can be reduced.

d. Made of such materials that are not easily destroyed by dogs, cats, pigs, and rats. Wood and metal are satisfactory materials for containers. .

Refuse Collection

Where there is no public refuse collection system, a member of the family or a family helper regularly collects the accumulated refuse in the home for final disposal.

In communities with public refuse collection systems, refuse collection involves two procedures:

1. Pick-up or gathering refuse from houses, institutions, and other establishments

2. Transportation of the collected refuse to the final disposal rate.

Some important points to consider in refuse collection are :

1. Frequent collection of refuse, especially garbage is necessary for good sanitation.

2. A longer interval between collection creates problems of storage and foul odors for the homeowner.

3. It is necessary to cover the refuse in the vehicles during transportation to final disposal sites to prevent flies, minimize odors, and remove traveling "eye-sores".

4. It is important to have adequate and properly maintained collection carts, trucks or other vehicles to eliminate collection delays and complaints from the inhabitants.

5. The route to the final disposal should be as direct as possible from the point of origin. However, it should preferably not pass busy streets.

6. Because of the nature of the waste materials, it is preferable to have collection done at night.

Refuse Disposal

The sanitary disposal of refuse needs closer attention both by the homeowner and by authorities concerned when there is an existing public refuse collection and disposal system.

In homes, the refuse disposal methods include:

a. Burial - Refuse deposited in pits and covered with soil. The most frequent defect on this method as practiced in our homes is the inadequate soil cover, making possible the excavation of the buried refuse by dogs, cats, and other animals.

b. Burning -This involves open burning on the ground and sometimes simple incinerators are used. In cities and other crowded communities.

c. Feeding to animals - Leftover foods and other garbage materials can be made use of by feeding to pigs, chickens, and other poultry and livestock.

d. Composting - Where garbage is not fed to animals and poultry, it may be composted, and the material used as soil conditioner and fertilizer. The simplest home composting method involves the deposition of garbage, leaves, other yard rubbish and animal manure into a pit and covered with soil, about two to three feet thick.

e. Grinding and disposal to sewer -There are now commercially available machines known as "garbage grinders." These are attached to the kitchen sink. Leftover foods, including small bones, are ground into smaller particles and washed down into the waste-water pipes and finally into the septic tank or public sewage collection system. This is a very satisfactory and convenient method of disposing garbage.

f. Sanitary landfill - Also known as the "cut and cover," it was developed in na effort to overcome the objections to the unsanitary open dump. It is a method of refuse disposal developed because of the many defects of open dumping encountered in practice. In a sanitary landfill, there is a systematic excavation of the soil, deposition of the refuse, covering with soil and compaction of the soil cover. Mechanized equipment such as bulldozers and cranes are used to advantage.

Recycling

Recycling is the recovery and reuse of any waste material where reusable materials are more available cheaply than fresh supplies of the same materials. The recycling principle is finding wider application in the conservation of the world's natural resources and in solving the problems of the wastes of a manufacturing process such as the remelting and recasting of metallic turning and off cuts is commonplace in industry.

Recycling is also the recovery and reprocessing for reuse of "discarded" materials, such as waste paper, scraped metals, and used glass bottles. The burning of garbage to produce electricity and the extraction of pure water from sewage and others are examples of recycling.

Recycling of material

Recycling waste and used material for some useful purpose is an effective means of conserving resources, of reducing waste disposal, and often eliminating cost.

For economic reasons, industries, reuse much of the scrap materials generated at their facilities. Some demolition materials and a larger amount of scrap of metal from automobiles are recycled. A small but increasing amount of residential and commercial wastes is currently recycled.

Chapter - 19

Health Effects related to Overweight and Obesity

Overweight and obesity may raise your risk for certain health problems and may be linked to certain emotional and social problems.

What are some health risks of overweight and obesity?

Type 2 diabetes

Type 2 diabetes is a disease that occurs when your blood glucose, also called blood sugar, is too high. About 8 out of 10 people with type 2 diabetes are overweight or have obesity. Over time, high blood glucose leads to problems such as heart disease, stroke, kidney disease, eye problems, nerve damage, and other health problems.

If you are at risk for type 2 diabetes, losing 5 to 7 percent of your body weight and getting regular physical activity may prevent or delay the onset of type 2 diabetes.

High blood pressure

High blood pressure, also called hypertension, is a condition in which blood flows through your blood vessels with a force greater than normal. High blood pressure can strain your heart, damage blood vessels, and raise your risk of heart attack, stroke, kidney disease, and death.

Overweight and obesity may raise your risk for certain health problems such as high blood pressure.

Heart disease

Heart disease is a term used to describe several problems that may affect your heart. If you have heart disease, you may have a heart attack, heart failure, sudden cardiac death, angina NIH external link, or an abnormal heart rhythm. High blood pressure, abnormal levels of blood fats, and high blood glucose levels may raise your risk for heart disease. Blood fats, also called blood lipids, include HDL cholesterol, LDL cholesterol, and triglycerides.

Stroke

Stroke is a condition in which the blood supply to your brain is suddenly cut off, caused by a blockage or the bursting of a blood vessel in your brain or neck. A stroke can damage brain tissue and make you unable to speak or move parts of your body. High blood pressure is the leading cause of strokes.

Sleep apnea

Sleep apnea is a common disorder in which you do not breathe regularly while sleeping. You may stop breathing altogether for short periods of time. Untreated sleep apnea may raise your risk of other health problems, such as type 2 diabetes and heart disease.

Metabolic syndrome

Metabolic syndrome is a group of conditions that put you at risk for heart disease, diabetes, and stroke. These conditions are

- high blood pressure

- high blood glucose levels

- high triglyceride levels in your blood

- low levels of HDL cholesterol (the "good" cholesterol) in your blood

- too much fat around your waist

Fatty liver diseases

Fatty liver diseases are conditions in which fat builds up in your liver. Fatty liver diseases include non-alcoholic fatty liver disease (NAFLD) and non-alcoholic steato-hepatitis (NASH). Fatty liver diseases may lead to severe liver damage, cirrhosis, or even liver failure.

Osteoarthritis

Osteoarthritis is a common, long-lasting health problem that causes pain, swelling, and reduced motion in your joints. Being overweight or having obesity may raise your risk of getting osteoarthritis by putting extra pressure on your joints and cartilage.

Gallbladder diseases

Overweight and obesity may raise your risk of getting gallbladder diseases, such as gallstones and cholecystitis. Imbalances in substances that make up bile cause gallstones. Gallstones may form if bile contains too much cholesterol.

Some cancers

Cancer NIH external link is a collection of related diseases. In all types of cancer, some of the body's cells begin to divide without stopping and spread into surrounding tissues. Overweight and obesity may raise your risk of developing certain types of cancer NIH external link.

Kidney disease

Kidney disease means that your kidneys are damaged and can't filter blood like they should. Obesity raises the risk of diabetes and high blood pressure, the most common causes of kidney disease. Even if you don't have diabetes or high blood pressure, obesity itself may promote kidney disease and quicken its progress.

Pregnancy problems

Overweight and obesity raise the risk of health problems that may occur during pregnancy. Pregnant women who are overweight or obese may have a greater chance of

- developing gestational diabetes

- having preeclampsia—high blood pressure during pregnancy, which can cause severe health problems for mother and baby if left untreated

- needing a cesarean section NIH external link, or C-section and, as a result, taking longer to recover after giving birth

What emotional and social problems are linked to overweight and obesity?

Overweight and obesity are associated with mental health problems such as depression NIH external link. People who deal with overweight and obesity may also be the subject of weight bias and stigma from others, including health care providers. This can lead to feelings of rejection, shame, or guilt—further worsening mental health problems.

Chapter - 20

Global Issues around Physical Activity

Physical inactivity is an issue that needs to be addressed on a global scale. It is a problem that affects countries regardless of income and is poised to have an increasingly negative impact on rates of obesity, non-communicable disease, and overall health. In order to understand physical inactivity at a systemic level, it's important to understand the global issues at play.

Global Determinants of Physical Activity

Several worldwide trends are thought to have a negative impact on physical activity participation.

Population Ageing

As life expectancy increases and fertility rates decline, the world's population is experiencing an unprecedented rise in adults aged 60 and older. With this trend has come an increased burden of non-communicable diseases that typically develop in middle and old ages. Despite the positive impact of physical activity (PA) on ageing and the prevention of chronic conditions, such as type 2 diabetes and heart diseases, older adults represent the least physically active age group. This trend is especially true in industrialised nations where both occupational and leisure time PA may be limited.

From an ecological perspective, the barriers to physical activity in older adults are varied. On an individual level, impaired physical & cognitive function and low perceived importance pose barriers to participation.[5] Obstacles at the social/cultural level include limited social support, lack of employment/volunteer opportunities, economic insecurity, and non-conducive cultural norms. The built environment, climate & seasonal changes, and transportation represent environmental/policy barriers that may have increased weight for older adults.

Urbanisation

Over the past 50 years, large segments of the global population have experienced rapid urbanisation. Urbanisation often entails violence, high-density traffic, low air quality, and pollution. In many places, these problems are also accompanied by a lack of sidewalks and poor access to parks and other sports/recreation facilities. Taken together, many experts posit that the environmental changes related to urban living discourage physical activity.

The evidence surrounding these assumptions is mixed. **Assah et al** found that living in an urban area was associated with lower levels of physical activity energy expenditure and a higher prevalence of metabolic syndrome compared to rural dwelling adults in Cameroon. Similar differences in physical activity were found in urban versus rural dwelling minors in the United States, and female adolescents in Portugal. Other studies have demonstrated no or an inverse relationship between PA & the degree of urbanisation. Perhaps in areas where rural life continues to entail strenuous domestic & occupational activities and urban planning has had little regard for encouraging active lifestyles, intuitive assumptions about the effects of urbanisation hold true; however, care should be taken to not extend such generalisations to countries or regions in which these conditions do not apply.

Mechanisation

Mechanisation is the process of replacing manual labor with machinery. Although technology can improve task efficiency, personal safety, and ease of mobility, it also minimises the physical effort required for self-transport and the performance of occupational and domestic activities. In doing so, mechanisation may inadvertently contribute to declining physical activity levels in the case that commensurate increases in leisure time PA do not take place.

Gender Equality

Men are more physically active than women across all age groups.[1] Findings from **Balish et al** suggest that levels of female empowerment, or gender equality, may play a role is this population pattern. Specifically, study results indicated that women living in countries with high gender equality were more likely to participate in leisure time PA than their counterparts living in countries with low gender equality. Interestingly, the same results were true for men. The authors hypothesised that increased female empowerment results in later marriages, delayed childbearing, and decreased overall birth rate. In turn, these changes allow both genders to invest moretime in leisure time PA for their children and themselves.

However, even in countries with high gender equality, differences in the needs of men and women exist. Particularly in the case of outdoor activities, living alone, fear of sexual assault, fear of verbal harassment,insecurities regarding body image, and familial time constraints more negatively influence participation in physical activity among women compared to men. Consequently, physical activity promotion among women should account for their unique concerns as well as the social, cultural, and religious norms that may engender them.

Climate Change

At present, cold, extreme heat and precipitation are all associated with reduced physical activity. Over time, global warming is poised to play a growing influence on physical activity levels. Rising temperatures may decrease physical inactivity in locations affected by cold climate.[22] On the other hand, an increase in physical inactivity is projected in locations that already experience high temperatures. For these high temperature regions, further decreases in physical activity have devastating implications for population health and should be accounted for in factoring the costs of climate change and the justification for mitigation efforts.

Future Directions

Going forward the **World Health Organization** recommends national level adoption of global physical activity guidelines, that should then be adapted to country-specific contexts. Apart from the global issues mentioned previously, the following factors should be considered on a regional/local basis:

- Social norms
- Language
- Religious values
- Security situation
- Geography
- Existing infrastructure
- Local government leadership

Existing patterns in physical activity

Perhaps the greatest need for future directions is the improved surveillance of physical activity worldwide. Particularly in low- and middle-income countries, data regarding levels of physical activity is limited. Such data is essential for tailoring global physical activity promotion to population specific needs/trends.

Chapter - 21

Why we Need to Stop Judging Mental Illness?

One in five adults in the U.S.—around 47.6 million people—experience mental illness. Less than half seek treatment. And those who do often wait a decade or more to get help. A full 20 percent of us are struggling with some form of mental illness...right now. And, most of us won't ask for help because we're embarrassed or ashamed.

When someone has a physical illness like cancer, diabetes or even a broken leg, we rally around them and offer support. Research has shown that having a strong support network can promote resilience and help people manage stress during difficult times.

So why is it that when someone is struggling with mental illness, from the mildest to the most severe forms, rather than offering support, we throw out tantrums like "Just be positive," or "A lot of people have it worse than you"? This emotional pain can do much more harm than good.

Misconceptions of Mental Illness are still widespread

There are many reasons why people develop mental health conditions and research suggests multiple overlapping causes. Genetics, biology, lifestyle, traumatic life events, or environmental injustice can all play a role. But regardless of the reason, mental health conditions are real health problems.

Stigmatization of mental illness isn't something new. Marginalization of people with mental illness has been going on for thousands of years. Early beliefs about the causes of mental illness, such as demonic possession, magic, the wrath of a deity or moral punishment, provoked reactions of fear, mistrust, and discrimination.

We've learned a lot about the nature of various psychological conditions since ancient times thanks to scientific advancements, yet people with mental illnesses continue to be perceived as violent, unpredictable, or dangerous. Inaccurate portrayals of mental illness in television, films, and other forms of media further perpetuate these beliefs.

According to clinical psychologist Todd Essig, Ph.D., there's a reason why we stigmatize. It's a kind of coping mechanism, albeit a flawed one. The idea behind this way of thinking is that if you create a wide gap between the mentally ill and those who are not ill, that distance almost creates a buffer, like you're safe because you're on the right side of the gap. But here's the reality: there is no wide gap; it's a fine line. And, anyone can become mentally ill at any time.

Another key issue is that some forms of mental illness are confused with personality traits, mischaracterized, or perceived as character defects rather than bona fide medical conditions.

To add to that, an abundance of positive thinking mantras, and inspirational quotes can give the impression that mental illness is just a mood or mindset that can be treated without a more serious healthcare intervention, such as medicine, talk therapy, and cognitive behavioral therapy.

Why Stigma Matters?

Hanging on to stigmas has some far-reaching effects—not just for the person experiencing mental illness, but for everyone.

It literally makes people sick

People who feel ashamed of their illness try to hide it and don't get the help they need. This means not only does their mental illness not get better, but their physical health can be impacted too. Case in point: research suggests that people with depression have a 40 percent higher risk of developing cardiovascular and metabolic diseases than the general population.

The stigma of mental illness can make relationships difficult to maintain. Family and friends may distance themselves, increasing feelings of isolation. It's a vicious cycle—loneliness can aggravate anxiety and depression and even trigger an inflammatory response that puts our immune system at risk.

It complicates treatment

Societal stigma can get in the way of how you're treated. Healthcare providers, unfortunately, are not immune to stereotypes. Studies have shown that people with a history of mental illness receive poorer quality care for their physical health problems and are often not taken seriously when describing their symptoms for non-mental health concerns.

It has a major economic impact

According to the World Economic Forum, mental illness will alone account for more than half of the global economic burden from non-communicable diseases between 2011–2030. A big part of that economic burden is the loss of income due to unemployment. The true costs may even be higher when you consider how mental illness ups the risk for things like cardiovascular disease, respiratory disease, and diabetes.

What we can do about it?

Sharing personal experiences is a powerful way to shift attitudes. In recent years, celebrities and sports figures have stepped forward to speak out about their own struggles with mental health issues and it's made huge strides in normalizing the conversation around mental health and spreading knowledge. Putting a face to mental illness and demonstrating that it can affect anyone, inspires others to open up about their issues.

Chapter - 22

Mental Health in Schools

Mental health awareness is an important issue for all educators, who are often the first line of defense for their students. Education professionals have recognized the impact that a student's mental health has on learning and achievement, and they realize that there's a great deal that can be done to help students with mental health issues. As a high school teacher with more than 23 years of experience, I welcome the fact that mental health awareness is finally becoming an important part of a school's function and curriculum.

Seeing the Signs in a Student

A few years ago, a student in my senior class changed drastically in a short period of time. I noticed that she no longer did her homework, and she didn't even try on her essays. Previously meticulous in her appearance, she would come to school disheveled, wearing the same clothes. When I tried to speak to her, she was uncharacteristically distant and withdrawn. Because I had some training in mental health awareness, I knew she was in some sort of trouble.

Luckily, my school had social workers on staff who could speak to her and assess her issues. They discovered that she was depressed and suicidal, and she needed immediate help. She was hospitalized for a period of time, but she was able to return to her classroom a few months later. With the help of medication and therapy, she managed to graduate with her class.

Understanding the Impact

The **National Alliance on Mental Illness** estimates that one in five people live with some sort of mental disorder or disease. Despite the fact that the average age of early signs of mental illness is 14, most individuals don't seek help until adulthood. Underlining the seriousness is the fact that 60 percent of high school students with mental illness don't graduate.

New York mental health experts recognized that earlier intervention could result in more positive outcomes for these students. Beginning in July 2018, New York will be the first state in the nation to require mental health education for all students. The overall mission of **New York's School Mental Health (SMH)** program is to promote healthy social, emotional, and behavioral development of students, and "break down barriers to learning so the general well-being of students, families, and school staff can be enhanced in collaboration with other comprehensive student support and services."

The SMH program supports the emotional health and academic growth of all students with the following:

- Integrating comprehensive services and support throughout every grade level

- Assessing mental health needs through universal, selective, and targeted interventions

- Providing access to behavioral and mental health services and programs

- Leveraging higher-level personnel, such as those working with the Department of Education, for necessary support and services

- Building collaborative relationships between the school and students' families and communities

Spreading Awareness across the Nation

Until mental health education is a mandatory aspect of all schools, teachers and administrators can work to promote awareness with their students. The key elements include the concept of self-care and responsibility for one's own mental health and wellness, with an emphasis on the fact that mental health is an integral part of health, and the concept of recovery from mental illness.

Teachers and students should be provided with ways to recognize signs of developing mental health problems, and there should be opportunities around the awareness and management of mental health crises, including the risk of suicide or self-harm. Further, instruction should address the relationship between mental health, substance abuse, and other negative coping behaviors, as well as the negative impact of stigma and cultural attitudes toward mental illness.

Because students spend most of their day at school, it just makes sense to have mental health awareness and education become part of the curriculum. When we empower students with knowledge, and encourage dialogue, students will be able to get the help they need.

Chapter - 23

If Health is Wealth, Why do we Ignore Mental Health?

Kathmandu, Nepal — For the past 20 years, Geeta tried everything to cure her son. She sold precious family ornaments and her prized gold chain; she took him to faith healers, temples, and astrologists across India; and she even married him off.

But nothing worked. Ramesh, 45, continued to remain elusive: He talked to no one but himself; he was socially withdrawn; and was often delusional, seeing things that no one else could.

"I tried everything but nothing worked," said Geeta, who lives in rural Bangalore, the capital city of Karnataka, a state in southern India. "I felt that an evil spirit had done black magic on him. I was fearful of being at home with just him. It's very sad because the community treats us badly."

But earlier this year, Geeta and Ramesh finally got some answers. Ramesh was diagnosed with chronic schizophrenia and put on anti-psychotic medication. Ramesh was connected with the public healthcare system after a community health worker recognized his symptoms. She referred him to a nearby primary healthcare center, eventually connecting him with a psychiatrist.

It was not an easy task. Nagaveni, a community health worker, recalled visiting the family "four or five times because they believed it was black magic."

"They weren't having any success with faith healers so they agreed."

But while it's early days, the intervention seems to have hit its mark. After all her efforts failed, Geeta said she is hopeful the medication will help her son. "He's my only son, I'm worried about his future. I want him to get better."

Mental Health neglected

An estimated 150 million people across India are in need of mental health care interventions, both short and long-term, according to India's latest **National Mental Health Survey 2015-16.** The survey, which was carried out across 12 states, found that the overall prevalence for current mental health morbidity was 10.6 percent.

Despite the high number of people who need care, mental health has been sorely neglected in India, rooted in stigma, taboo, and myths.

Poor awareness about the symptoms of mental illness, stigma and the lack of mental health services available has resulted in a massive treatment gap, with inadequate numbers of trained mental health care professionals. The survey found that, depending on the state, between 70 and 92 percent of those in need of mental health care failed to receive any treatment.

There are just 0.3 psychiatrists, 0.07 psychologists and 0.07 social workers per 100,000 people in India. To compare, the ratio of psychiatrists in developed countries is 6.6 per 100,000 and the average number of mental hospitals globally is 0.04 per 100,000 while it's only 0.004 in India.

Community Mental Healthcare

The lack of mental health care workers is hardly a new, or ignored, issue. In 1982, the government of India began implementing its **National**

Mental Health Program with the broader aim of integrating mental health care with general care. Fourteen years later, the program expanded to the district level with the vision that each of India's 630 districts would have a **District Mental Health Program** by 2025.

The objective of the DMHP is to provide community mental health services at the primary health care level by training a mental health team comprised of a psychiatrist, psychologist, psychiatric social workers, and nurses in each district, along with increasing awareness and reducing stigma.

But roll out has been slow. As of 2015, nearly two decades after the program launched, it was only prevalent in 27 percent of districts. The DMHP has also been plagued by inaccessible funding and administrative and programmatic problems such as poor governance, unrealistic expectations from low paid and poorly motivated health care workers, and a lack of understanding of ground realities.

But perhaps the chief shortfall has been its inability to fill the required number of professionals required in each district.

Recognizing this, staff from the **National Institute of Mental Health** and **Neuro Sciences** and the **government of Karnataka,** in southwest India, realized that community health workers, better known as **Accredited Social Health Activists, or ASHA** workers, presented a unique opportunity to fill the gap. Starting in 2016, they began giving the workers extra training in identifying and dealing with mental health issues.

There are more than 800,000 ASHA workers across India who act as interface between the community and public health system. The workers are specially trained local women, selected from those between the ages of 25 and 45 who have completed 10th grade schooling. Based in villages, their roles include counselling women on pregnancy, safe delivery, and breastfeeding, facilitating immunizations, and diabetes checks amid other health-related services.

"We have thirty districts in Karnataka and apart from the urban areas, we won't find psychiatrists, psychologists or any other mental health professionals," said Anish Cherian, from the department of psychiatric social work at NIMHANS, who is involved with the program. "There's a huge skill shortage and the distribution of professionals hasn't been even."

As a result, Karnataka has trained more than 22,000 workers on basic mental health in the last year alone. The training is just one day, and is carried out by each district's DMHP and then continued one day per month by medical officers.

The ongoing training includes teaching ASHA workers how to recognize common to severe mental health problems like schizophrenia, anxiety, depression, and alcohol abuse along with teaching them how to refer patients to a professional at the primary health care level and also to provide basic counselling.

Cherian explained that because most cases require basic interventions such as listening, talking, and minor lifestyle changes, he said ASHA workers were in a unique position to offer such services in a supportive way.

"Most cases need basic interventions. Many people have tension, fatigue, and body aches and pains. They just need someone to talk to, to sit with them and support them," he said.

A psychiatrist for Bangalore DMHP, Dr. Chetan Kumar, said utilizing ASHA workers was about strengthening the system rather than creating a new one. "Increasing the number of psychologists and psychiatrists alone won't help — that would take another 150 years to fill the gap," he said.

But for patients with more severe mental health illnesses like Ramesh, linkage to care is a long road because of the lack of providers. Patients in rural areas who need care often have to travel more than 100 kilometers to see a psychiatrist, Cherian said.

Structural issues

The use of ASHA workers for India's mental health response is not just confined to Karnataka.

In the northern Indian state of Madhya Pradesh, ESSENCE, a five-year research project that began last year by Harvard Medical School and Sangath, an NGO in south India in partnership with the state government, is evaluating the use of technology interventions to train and support ASHA workers to deliver therapy for depression.

Such efforts are part of India's broader plan to implement its first ever National Mental Health Policy which was launched in 2014. The policy aims to provide universal access to mental health care by enhancing understanding of mental health. The policy called for increased funding along with an increased number of professionals to be trained on all levels from the community to specialized psychiatrists.

Much of the policy is reliant on individual states to implement it effectively. It is widely acknowledged that southern states like Karnataka are more likely to spend funds more efficiently on district-level programs than relatively poorer and more populous states in the north.

Greg Armstrong, research fellow at the Centre for Mental Health at the University of Melbourne, Australia, said the use of ASHA workers to provide basic mental health care was encouraging as it signaled India was moving closer to being able to fulfil the human right of access to mental health treatment.

Last year, the country passed the Mental Health Care Act 2017, which looks to empower people suffering from mental illness and to safeguard their rights and access to treatment without discrimination, amid other clauses.

Armstrong stressed that while ASHA workers could fill a gap in the system, they were simultaneously creating demand for treatment when specialized supply was not yet fully available.

"ASHAs have to do everything and now we're getting them to do mental health care. It's not a bad thing but it creates a lot of pressure when the nearest psychiatrist might be six hours away," he said. "We need to consider the whole mental health system on a region-by-region or district-by-district basis."

So, while on paper 27 percent of India's districts have a district mental health program, many are lacking a fully equipped team.

To this end, Armstrong highlighted that many mental health problems including depression may in many cases be strongly intertwined with major structural and social issues such as entrenched poverty, domestic violence, and early marriage. Armstrong said this meant there was an imperative to not to drop vigilance in addressing broader issues in India.

Looking ahead, experts are encouraged that momentum is building in India to provide better care and combat stigma. But it's a long road.

"It's a mammoth task," Dr Kumar said. "Indians aren't immune to mental health illnesses but they don't believe they suffer from it."

Chapter - 24

Overcoming the Taboo of Mental Health in India amidst the Pandemic - Hemant Sethi

The topics of mental health, social isolation and anxiety over the loss of employment have never been in greater focus than in the age of COVID-19. The fact that mental illnesses can lead to serious adverse outcomes if neglected, makes it even more important to recognize and address this problem during these times of the pandemic. The **World Health Organization (WHO)** stated in a report that suicides due to depression are the second-most common cause of death in individuals aged 15 to 29 years of age. This busts the myth that the illness only adversely affects the elderly. Going by the report, anyone, whether young or old, could become a victim of depression or other mental illnesses. However, the subject of mental illness is not one that most people would want to talk about openly, and even less, accept the fact that they may be suffering from this problem. This outlook needs to change.

Covid-19 and mental illnesses

Mental ailments can stem from several causative factors. The death of a loved one, or the loss of one's employment. Factors such as long-term stress, solitude, the fear of poverty, and losing one's source of income are some of the more common reasons for debilitating mental ailments in individuals. The **Covid-19 pandemic** has amplified these circumstances, impacting many people.

According to a study published in the Indian Journal of Psychiatry, on the prevalence of psychological morbidities among the general population, healthcare workers, and COVID-19 patients, about half of the population faced psychological impacts of the COVID-19 pandemic. Poor sleep quality (40%), stress (34%), and psychological distress (34%) were the most reported problems across various studies. The report also mentions another online Indian survey which found that about 40.5% of the participants reported anxiety or depressive symptoms. About three-fourths (74.1%) of the participants reported a moderate level of stress, and 71.7% reported poor well-being.

The taboo of mental illness in India

A report states that as per WHO 7.5 percent of Indians suffer from some mental disorder and predicts that by the end of this year roughly 20 percent of India will suffer from mental illnesses. It estimates that about 56 million Indians suffer from depression and another 38 million Indians suffer from anxiety disorders. However, India seems to be far behind in terms of identifying and addressing mental health and the issues related to it.

Depression and anxiety attacks are frequently tagged as minor inconveniences only faced by the uber-rich. What's worse, Individuals with mental conditions tend to hide their issues due to fear of being looked down upon and judged by a conservative society. Shedding these negative qualities and bringing about a culture change across the board may take several years in India.

Overcoming the taboo of mental illness

On the bright side, here are some examples of how public bodies and organisations can help those with existing mental health conditions. Using these workarounds, eventually, the taboos associated with mental ailments in India can be eliminated.

Increasing the number of mental health experts

There is a serious dearth of mental health professionals in the country. On the surface, it seems that India's youngsters do not find the field of mental healthcare as exciting or financially rewarding as, say, software engineering or chartered accountancy. As a result, there are simply not enough experts in the country who can provide professional help to the millions, who suffer from such conditions daily. As a solution, students can be encouraged from a young age to pursue a career in psychiatry or other specialised mental health practices. The government can introduce schemes that make it easier for people to get into such courses and graduate with minimal fuss.

On an organisational level, the main management team could increase the number of mental health experts within the company premises. The presence of more professionals can positively influence the way your workers deal with their mental health conditions arising from job stress or other, more personal reasons.

Providing greater access to treatments

Conditions such as depression, schizophrenia and anxiety need expert attention and treatment that cannot be provided by a general physician or even a common psychiatrist. Often, treatments for such conditions may be a complex and drawn-out process and beyond affordability for common people. As a result, several people with such conditions may continue to live through their illnesses.

Delaying or denying treatment to people who need it most may be the reason for countless deaths across the age and region spectrum. To avoid such a snowballing of bad things, the government could make mental healthcare more affordable and accessible for individuals regardless of their economic status. The Healthcare Act, introduced in 2017, is a positive step in this direction.

Building mental fortitude through empathy

Businesses should ensure they have a proper communication channel through which workers with mental health conditions can get through to qualified counselors or designated health experts. The privacy of an individual suffering from a mental health condition is vital and must be respected and preserved. Empathy must be shown towards employees who are stressed with their work or show signs of depression. Occupational safety training should also include proper ways to treat work colleagues in a shared workplace regardless of whether they have mental illnesses or not. Behaviour-based safety programs can be nicely complemented by mental health training and monitoring.

Needless to say, such empathy must also be demonstrated by people across the country towards their fellow citizens. While it may not be fair to expect a massive shift in people's perceptions regarding mental health and wellness, even small changes in behaviour and attitude will go a long way in alleviating the mental health and well-being of a lot of people.

The author is Country Head, British Safety Council, India. Views expressed are personal and do not reflect the official position or policy of the Financial Express Online.

Chapter - 25

How do Thoughts and Emotions Affect Health?

Your thoughts and emotions can affect your health. Emotions that are freely experienced and expressed without judgment or attachment tend to flow fluidly without impacting our health. On the other hand, repressed emotions (especially fearful or negative ones) can zap mental energy, negatively affect the body, and lead to health problems..

It's important to recognize our thoughts and emotions and be aware of the effect they have—not only on each other, but also on our bodies, behavior, and relationships.

Poorly-managed negative emotions are not good for your health

Negative attitudes and feelings of helplessness and hopelessness can create chronic stress, which upsets the body's hormone balance, depletes the brain chemicals required for happiness, and damages the immune system. Chronic stress can actually decrease our lifespan.

Poorly managed or repressed anger (hostility) is also related to a slew of health conditions, such as hypertension (high blood pressure), cardiovascular disease, digestive disorders, and infection.

The Importance of Positive Emotions

Scientist Barbara Fredrickson has shown that positive emotions:

- Broaden our perspective of the world (thus inspiring more creativity, wonder, and options)

- Build over time, creating lasting emotional resilience and flourishing.

Dr. Fredrickson has spent years researching and publishing the physical and emotional benefits of positivity, including faster recovery from cardiovascular stress, better sleep, fewer colds, and a greater sense of overall happiness. The good news is not only that positive attitudes—such as playfulness, gratitude, awe, love, interest, serenity, and feeling connected to others—have a direct impact on health and wellbeing, but that we can develop them ourselves with practice.

Overcoming our negativity bias

Because we are wired to defend against threat and loss in life, we tend to prioritize bad over good. While this is a tidy survival mechanism for someone who needs to stay hyper vigilant in a dangerous environment, the truth is that for most of us, this "negativity bias" is counter-productive.

Our "negativity bias" means that we spend too much time ruminating over the minor frustrations we experience—bad traffic or a disagreement with a loved one— and ignore the many chances we have to experience wonder, awe, and gratitude throughout the day.

In order to offset this negativity bias and experience a harmonious emotional state, Fredrickson proposes that we need to experience three positive emotions for every negative one. This, she claims, can be done intentionally for those of us less "wired" to positivity. These positive emotions literally reverse the physical effects of negativity and build up psychological resources that contribute to a flourishing life.

The Role of Forgiveness

Forgiveness means fully accepting that a negative event has occurred and relinquishing our negative feelings surrounding the circumstance. Research shows that forgiveness helps us experience better mental, emotional and physical health.

- 70% reported a decrease in their feelings of hurt

- 13% experienced reduced anger

- 27% experienced fewer physical complaints (for example, pain, gastrointestinal upset, dizziness, etc.)

The practice of forgiveness has also been linked to better immune function and a longer lifespan. Other studies have shown that forgiveness has more than just a metaphorical effect on the heart: it can actually lower our blood pressure and improve cardiovascular health as well.

The Benefits of Gratitude

Ten ways to be a more thankful personBrene Brown discusses the relationship between joy and gratitude Acknowledging the good aspects of life and giving thanks have a powerful impact on emotional wellbeing. In a landmark study, people who were asked to count their blessings felt happier, exercised more, had fewer physical complaints, and slept better than those who created lists of hassles.

Brené Brown has found that there is a relationship between joy and gratitude, but with a surprising twist: It's not joy that makes us grateful, but gratitude that makes us joyful.

Positive emotions lead to emotional resilience

Positive emotions have a scientific purpose—to help the body recover from the ill effects of persistent negative emotions. Thus cultivating positivity over time can help us become more resilient in the face of crisis or stress.

Emotional resilience is like a rubber band—no matter how far a resilient person is stretched or pulled by negative emotions, he or she has the ability to bounce back to his or her original state.

Resilient people are able to experience tough emotions like pain, sorrow, frustration, and grief without falling apart. Resilient people do not deny the pain or suffering they are experiencing; rather, they retain a sense of positivity that helps them overcome the negative effects of their situation. In fact, some people are able to look at challenging times with optimism and hope, knowing that their hardships will lead to personal growth and an expanded outlook on life.

Chapter - 26

Physical Activity Is Good for the Mind and the Body

Everyone has their own way to "recharge" their sense of well-being — something that makes them feel good physically, emotionally, and spiritually even if they aren't consciously aware of it. Personally, I know that few things can improve my day as quickly as a walk around the block or even just getting up from my desk and doing some push-ups. A hike through the woods is ideal when I can make it happen. But that's me. It's not simply that I enjoy these activities but also that they literally make me feel better and clear my mind.

Mental health and physical health are closely connected. No kidding — what's good for the body is often good for the mind. Knowing what you can do physically that has this effect for you will change your day and your life.

Physical activity has many well-established mental health benefits. These are published in the **Physical Activity Guidelines** for Americans and include improved brain health and cognitive function (the ability to think, if you will), a reduced risk of anxiety and depression, and improved sleep and overall quality of life. Although not a cure-all, increasing physical activity directly contributes to improved mental health and better overall health and well-being.

Learning how to routinely manage stress and getting screened for depression are simply good prevention practices. Awareness is especially critical at this time of year when disruptions to healthy habits and choices can be more likely and more jarring. Shorter days and colder temperatures have a way of interrupting routines — as do the holidays, with both their joys and their stresses. When the plentiful sunshine and clear skies of temperate months give way to unpredictable weather, less daylight, and festive gatherings, it may happen unconsciously or seem natural to be distracted from being as physically active. However, that tendency is precisely why it's so important that we are ever more mindful of our physical and emotional health — and how we can maintain both — during this time of year.

Roughly half of all people in the United States will be diagnosed with a mental health disorder at some point in their lifetime, with anxiety and anxiety disorders being the most common. Major depression, another of the most common mental health disorders, is also a leading cause of disability for middle-aged adults. Compounding all of this, mental health disorders like depression and anxiety can affect people's ability to take part in health-promoting behaviors, including physical activity. In addition, physical health problems can contribute to mental health problems and make it harder for people to get treatment for mental health disorders.

The COVID-19 pandemic has brought the need to take care of our physical and emotional health to light even more so these past 2 years. Recently, the U.S. Surgeon General highlighted how the pandemic has exacerbated the mental health crisis in youthThis link is external to health.gov..

The good news is that even small amounts of physical activity can immediately reduce symptoms of anxiety in adults and older adults. Depression has also shown to be responsive to physical activity. Research suggests that increased physical activity, of any kind, can improve

 Mental Health And Physical Health

depression symptoms experienced by people across the lifespan. Engaging in regular physical activity has also been shown to reduce the risk of developing depression in children and adults.

Though the seasons and our life circumstances may change, our basic needs do not. Just as we shift from shorts to coats or fresh summer fruits and vegetables to heartier fall food choices, so too must we shift our seasonal approach to how we stay physically active. Some of that is simply adapting to conditions: bundling up for a walk, wearing the appropriate shoes, or playing in the snow with the kids instead of playing soccer in the grass.

Sometimes there's a bit more creativity involved. Often this means finding ways to simplify activity or make it more accessible. For example, it may not be possible to get to the gym or even take a walk due to weather or any number of reasons. In those instances, other options include adding new types of movementThis link is external to health.gov. — such as impromptu dance parties at home — or doing a few household choresThis link is external to health.gov. (yes, it all counts as physical activity).

During the COVID-19 pandemic, I built a makeshift gym in my garage as an alternative to driving back and forth to the gym several miles from home. That has not only saved me time and money but also afforded me the opportunity to get 15 to 45 minutes of muscle-strengthening physical activity in at odd times of the day.

The point to remember is that no matter the approach, the Physical Activity Guidelines recommend that adults get at least 150 minutes of moderate-intensity aerobic activity (anything that gets your heart beating faster) each week and at least 2 days per week of muscle-strengthening activity (anything that makes your muscles work harder than usual). Youth need 60 minutes or more of physical activity each day. Preschool-aged children ages 3 to 5 years need to be active throughout the day — with adult caregivers encouraging active play — to enhance growth and development. Striving toward these goals and then continuing to get physical activity, in some shape or form, contributes to better health outcomes both immediately and over the long term.

For youth, sports offer additional avenues to more physical activity and improved mental health. Youth who participate in sports may enjoy psychosocial health benefits beyond the benefits they gain from other forms of leisure-time physical activity. Psychological health benefits include higher levels of perceived competence, confidence, and self-esteem — not to mention the benefits of team building, leadership, and resilience, which are important skills to apply on the field and throughout life. Research has also shown that youth sports participants have a reduced risk of suicide and suicidal thoughts and **tendencies**. Additionally, team sports participation during adolescence may lead to better mental health outcomes in adulthood (e.g., less anxiety and depression) for people exposed to adverse childhood experiences. In addition to the physical and mental health benefits, sports can be just plain fun.

Physical activity's implications for significant positive effects on mental health and social well-being are enormous, impacting every facet of life. In fact, because of this national imperative, the presidential executive order that re-established the President's Council on Sports, Fitness & NutritionThis link is external to health.gov. explicitly seeks to "expand national awareness of the importance of mental health as it pertains to physical fitness and nutrition." While physical activity is not a substitute for mental health treatment when needed and it's not the answer to certain mental health challenges, it does play a significant role in our emotional and cognitive well-being.

No matter how we choose to be active during the holiday season — or any season — every effort to move counts toward achieving recommended physical activity goals and will have positive impacts on both the mind and the body. Along with preventing diabetes, high blood pressure, obesity, and the additional risks associated with these co-morbidities, physical activity's positive effect on mental health is yet another important reason to be active and move your way.

Chapter - 27

Effects of Excess Stress on Physical and Mental Health

"It is extremely important to deal with stress as soon as possible, and not allow it to become chronic in nature." Ritika Aggarwal Mehta, consultant psychologist

A hectic lifestyle coupled with an erratic sleep pattern and certain situations can lead to stress.

"Stress is a response to a threat in any given situation. In other words, it triggers your body's 'fight-or-flight' response. This stress response helps protect the body in an emergency by preparing you to react quickly to the situation. However, when this stress response fires continuously and stress levels remain elevated over a long period of time, then this chronic stress can put your physical and mental wellbeing at risk," said Ritika Aggarwal Mehta, consultant psychologist, Jaslok Hospital and Research Center.

Given below, are the many effects of stress.

Physical health side-effects:

Respiratory: When stressed, we tend to breathe faster in an attempt to distribute oxygen-rich blood to the body. Some report feeling that they can't breathe or feel a heaviness in their chest. "This can exacerbate existing breathing issues and/ or may create anxiety and panic where one may believe one has a serious physical health issue," she explained.

Cardiovascular: Stress causes your heart to pump blood faster as well as the blood vessels to constrict so as to divert more oxygen to your muscles to give you the strength to fight off the trigger or flee from it. However, this also raises one's blood pressure. Frequent or chronic stress can increase one's risk of developing high BP, a stroke or heart attack.

Digestive: Stress increases the risk of acid reflux, ulcers, stomach aches and cramps, bloating, diarrhoea or constipation, nausea, and vomiting.

Muscular: To protect oneself from injury, the muscles tend to tighten for the duration of the stressful situation and relax thereafter. "If the stress becomes chronic, they don't get a chance to relax and this can cause headaches, back and shoulder pain, generalised body pain, and tiredness. This pain can cause further issues when one is unable to exercise due to it or has to take medication to deal with it," she said.

Immunity: Chronic stress tends to reduce one's ability to fight off infections making one more prone to infection and viral illnesses. It can also affect one's recovery time

Diabetes: The body, when stressed, tends to increase the production of glucose to give one the extra energy required. When the stress becomes chronic, the body may not be able to keep up and this increases the risk of developing type 2 diabetes.

Dental: Bruxism or teeth grinding can also be caused by stress which can affect one's dental health in the long run.

Sexuality and male reproductive health: Chronic stress can cause testosterone to start dropping which may affect sperm production, erectile dysfunction, or impotence. It can also increase the risk of infection to the reproductive organs. Chronic stress also tends to cause exhaustion which can lead to a loss of libido.

Sexuality and female reproductive health: Exhaustion can lead to a loss of libido for women as well. Additionally, it can affect the menstrual cycle – changes in menstrual regularity and flow and increased menstrual pain and cramps. If one is menopausal, chronic stress can enhance the physical symptoms.

Mental health side-effects:

Sleep: Stress tends to cause difficulty in falling asleep and staying asleep. It may also affect one's sleep cycle. Chronic stress can lead to insomnia.

Appetite: Stress tends to affect appetite wherein it may either increase or decrease.

Loss of control: Stress can cause one to feel overwhelmed and this can lead to one feeling one is losing control. This can further increase the feelings of stress

Mental health conditions: "Chronic stress can increase one's risk for depression, panic attacks, anxiety disorders, and substance use disorders. It can also cause irritation and increased anger outbursts when one finds it difficult to cope with the stressors," the expert told indianexpress.com.

Executive functions: "Stress may affect one's attention and concentration causing a task to take longer to complete."

"It can also impact memory as it becomes more difficult to create short term memories and transfer said short term memories to long term storage, making it more difficult to retain information and thus learn."

"The organisation of information also becomes difficult in view of multiple thoughts racing and interfering with one's thought process."

"Judgement can be affected."

"It is, therefore, extremely important to deal with stress as soon as possible, and not allow it to become chronic in nature. If you're finding it difficult to manage the stress, please reach out to a mental health practitioner who can help you work on coping with it better," she suggested.

Conclusion

Our physical, psychological and social stability requires mental health. It has an impact on how we think, feel and act. It also assists in deciding how we deal with stress, how we respond to others, and how we make choices. At all stages of life, mental health is essential, from infancy and adolescence through adulthood. Several factors contribute to mental health issues, including:

- Biological causes, such as genes or brain chemistry

- Childhood events, such as trauma or neglect and

- Family history of mental health problems.

Those with mental health issues can get help from a mental asylum in Pune, and many can fully recover.

Why is it important?

Good mental health is important for people to:

   Mental Health And Physical Health

- achieve their full potential
- dealing with life pressures
- function productively
- make significant contributions to their communities

Importance of Mental Health Treatment

Your emotional well-being is affecting everything about your life. It affects your relationships and your family. It impacts your work performance and your personal life. Not to mention, this affects your overall physical well-being tremendously.

Relationships & mental health: Some of the common mental illness symptoms include swings in mood, depression, intense feelings of frustration and other behaviours that can influence relationships. Family members are beginning to feel like they barely know you anymore, and relations are strained.

Mental health & career: The effects of mental illness will also make it hard to work in the workplace. People with depression, for example, also lack the motivation to be successful.

Mental health & physical health: There is a clear link between your mental well-being and your physical health. Those with impaired mental health, and vice versa, are more likely to suffer from chronic physical conditions.

How to Maintain your Mental well-being?

Whether you are dealing with your mental health or thinking like you might be able to do so, there are various things that you can do to be successful with your recovery or to get answers. The first is to speak to a medical professional about how you feel and your mental health issues. Your doctor can advise you to make a few adjustments to the lifestyle and see if they help before you turn to the medication. Medication is, therefore, important for certain citizens. There's no one-size-fits-all medication but figuring out what's right for you is about that. While there is no standardized approach to the treatment of mental illness, there are some widely accepted safe behavioural habits that improve one's mental health

- Exercising and becoming healthy
- Be social and interact with your loved ones

- Take up a new hobby and learn something new
- Be conscious and/or volunteer
- Get enough sleep
- Stop drugs and alcohol
- Build effective coping skills

Nevertheless, the stigma of mental illness will lead people to hide and stop doing the things needed to feel better. It's essential to be as diligent in taking care of your mental state as you are in taking care of your body when you're sick. And there is no harm in visiting a mental hospital in Pune and getting yourself checked.

What is Mental Health?

Sometimes people are not sure what mental health is and feel a bit afraid of it. Think about physical health. That doesn't have the same negative impact does it? Our physical health can be good or poor and it can vary from day to day. When our physical health is good we can enjoy life to the full.

At other times we can be unwell and this can last for weeks or months. Or we might be unwell just for a couple of days then we are back to normal. Sometimes our physical health is poor because we haven't taken good care of ourselves or because we were born with a tendency to certain illnesses. When we are unwell we are likely to have less energy and motivation and find taking part in work or play more difficult.

All of these things are true of mental health. The main difference between physical and mental health is that our emotions, our ability to work and our relationships are the main things to be influenced by our mental health.

When our mental health is positive we can cope with ups and downs. Our mood is stable and we feel optimistic. When we are mentally unwell we may experience mental or emotional pain. Our mood may be low and we might lose confidence in our ability to cope with life´s challenges. Sometimes we can have long term mental health problems, just as we can get longer lasting physical illnesses... and we can recover in much the same way.

Of course the other big difference is that you can´t get a mental health problem from someone else - it isn´t catching like the flu. Physical and mental health have an effect on each other. If your physical health is poor your mental health is likely to be low. If your mental health is poor you are more likely to get physically ill.

The good news is that you can make a difference to your own mental health. Scotland's Mental Health First Aid is one of the ways that helps you make a difference to your own and other people's mental health.

Link between Physical and Mental Health

The time when we used to think the mind and the body were entirely separate entities may be long gone, but few of us probably realise how closely linked they are when it comes to our health and wellbeing. Yet the evidence that physical health has a significant impact on mental health – and vice versa – is mounting up.

When we talk about health these days we no longer just mean health in a physical sense. According to the World Health Organization health is 'a state of complete physical, mental and social wellbeing and not merely the absence of disease or infirmity' (i). Indeed if you want to lead a happy, fulfilling life, it's important to be aware of how your physical health and fitness affect your mental health as well as why your state of mind is important for your physical wellbeing.

Today we know if you're living with a serious mental illness you have a higher risk of being affected by a range of chronic physical conditions too. Experts from the Kings Fund suggest 46 per cent of people with a mental health problem also have a long-term physical condition (ii). Scientists have also recently discovered people with more mental health problems may also age faster than the rest of the population (iii).

The opposite is also true: if you have a chronic physical health condition you're more likely to experience mental health issues such as anxiety and depression than if you were physically well. In fact, according to the Mental Health Foundation, almost one in three people with a long-term physical health condition also has a mental health problem (iv).

So, given that more than 15 million people in England alone are believed to have one or more long-term physical conditions – including diabetes, arthritis, asthma and cardiovascular disease – it should be no surprise that mental health problems in general are considered the largest single cause of disability in the UK, compared with specific physical illnesses such as cancer and heart disease (v).

Yet, if you have a physical health condition it doesn't automatically mean you'll experience mental illness too (or the other way around). Discovering how your wellbeing in one area can directly or indirectly affect the other could help you discover the steps you can take to stay as healthy as possible – both physically and mentally.

How physical health affects mental health?

If you're living with a long-term physical condition, in addition to physical symptoms and chronic pain you may also experience the emotional stress that comes with having to cope with your symptoms on a day-to-day basis. All of these things can lead to mental health problems such as depression and anxiety, not to mention feeling isolated and cut off from your social supports.

Having a chronic physical condition can also deplete your energy, which can mean you won't be as active as you should be. However not being physically active can have a negative impact on your mental well-being too (for more details see below).

Some of the physical conditions that can often co-exist with mental well-being issues include the following:

Psoriasis: This often debilitating skin condition is associated with high levels of stress, low self-esteem as well as depression, with those affected often experiencing problems with their quality of life. Read more about it in our psoriasis guide.

Diabetes: According to Diabetes UK, around four in 10 people with diabetes experience diabetes-related emotional distress, which can make it more difficult for them to manage their condition (vi). The charity also claims the variable blood glucose levels that are a feature of diabetes can cause feelings of anxiety of anger, while research suggests those with diabetes are twice as likely to experience depression than the rest of the population (vi).

Heart problems: The Centers for Disease Control in the US claims there's evidence to suggest mental health disorders such as depression, anxiety and post-traumatic stress disorder (PTSD) can develop in people who've had a cardiac event such as heart failure, stroke or heart attack (vii). It believes this may happen when heart patients experience pain, fear of death or disability, lack of confidence, anxiety and financial problems as a result of having their condition.

Parkinson's disease: People with Parkinson's often experience mental health issues alongside their physical symptoms, says Parkinson's UK (viii). Two of the most common health conditions affecting people with Parkinson's are anxiety and depression, with nearly half of those with Parkinson's experiencing one or the other. According to the charity, anxiety and depression can be triggered by the stress of receiving a diagnosis of the condition, as well as by physical changes in the brain caused by the condition itself.

Multiple sclerosis: According to the MS Society it's not unusual to experience depression, stress and anxiety if you have multiple sclerosis (MS), with up to half of people with the condition experiencing depression at some point (ix). Some of the factors that can contribute to mental health issues, says the charity, include nerve damage in the frontal lobe caused by MS as well as having to cope emotionally with a diagnosis of the condition. Certain medicines commonly used to treat MS and its related symptoms can also cause temporary mood and behaviour changes in some people (x).

Thyroid problems: Thyroid disorders, says the British Thyroid Foundation, often have mental as well as physical symptoms, most notably hyperthyroidism (overactive thyroid), hypothyroidism (underactive thyroidism), thyroid-related eye disease and thyroid cancer (xi). The charity cites anxiety, depression, mood swings, concentration difficulties, short-term memory lapses and lack of mental alertness as common thyroid-related emotional problems.

Why is physical fitness important for mental health?

Being physically active on a regular basis is good for your body in many ways. However it also helps maintain your mental health and wellbeing, with scientists believing exercise could play an important role in the management of mild to moderate mental health conditions, particularly depression and anxiety.

Physical activity can have a positive effect on your mood, particularly at times when you're feeling a bit low. It can help you deal with stress too, as well as boost your self-esteem and generally make you feel better in yourself. Why? Because physical activity is thought to release feel-good hormones that make you feel better in yourself overall. If you're not very physically fit, on the other hand, you could have an increased risk of experiencing mental health issues such as depression, anxiety or both, says a large-scale UK study . The results of the study found those who had low combined cardio-respiratory fitness and muscle strength were 98 per cent more likely to experience depression and 60 per cent more likely to experience anxiety compared with others who were physically fitter.

Mental health impacts on physical health

While many physical health conditions are associated with emotional and mental wellbeing problems, it's true that people living with mental illness tend to have a higher-than-average risk of being physically unwell too.

One possible explanation is that having a mental illness can sometimes make people adopt unhealthy habits, such as smoking, drinking too much alcohol or abusing drugs – all of which can have consequences for their physical health.

People with mental illness may also be less motivated to look after themselves physically compared with those who are mentally well. Similarly people living with mental ill health sometimes have higher rates of unemployment, housing insecurity and social isolation, any or all of which can also contribute to their vulnerability towards developing chronic physical conditions.

According to the **Mental Health Foundation**, people with mental health problems may be more likely to experience poor physical health because:

- They have genes that increase their risk of developing both mental and physical health problems.

- They may have difficulties with concentration and planning – this could, for instance, make it harder for them to arrange or attend appointments with doctors and other health professionals.

- They don't get the support they need to change unhealthy behaviours such as drinking and smoking, as it may be assumed they aren't capable of making such changes.

- They're less likely to get medical help because doctors may assume their physical symptoms are part of their mental illness. This could mean physical symptoms aren't investigated properly.

- They're also less likely to get routine tests such as blood pressure and cholesterol, which could help spot symptoms of physical conditions earlier.

Mental illness and cardiovascular disease

Mental ill health has been linked to a number of physical conditions including cancer, musculoskeletal problems such as back pain, irritable bowel syndrome (IBS), respiratory illnesses and several others including cardiovascular disease.

A study carried out by King's College London that followed more than 3.2 million people with severe mental illness showed they have a substantially increased risk for developing cardiovascular disease compared to the general population (xv).

In the study, those with illnesses such as schizophrenia, bipolar disorder and major depression were found to have a 53 per cent higher risk for cardiovascular disease than the general population, with a 78 per cent higher risk of developing cardiovascular disease in the long term. Their risk of dying from cardiovascular disease was also found to be 85 per cent higher than those of a similar age in the general population.

A scientific statement issued by the American Heart Association (xvi) also claims mental health problems can negatively impact your health and risk factors for heart disease and stroke. The statement adds that mental health conditions including depression, chronic stress, anxiety, anger, pessimism and dissatisfaction with life are associated with potentially harmful biological responses including:

- Irregular heart rate and rhythm

- Increased blood pressure

- Reduced blood flow to the heart

In a more positive light, researchers based at Duke University and the University of Michigan suggest treating mental health problems in young people could help them stay physically healthier in later life (iii).

They discovered that, during the 30-year study period, people with mental disorders were more likely to develop physical diseases plus they died earlier than those without mental health problems. The researchers conclude that getting prompt mental health care for young people who need it could help reduce the development of physical diseases in the same people when they're older.

How do you maintain physical and mental well-being?

If you have a physical health condition, it's not inevitable that you'll also develop a mental health illness, or vice versa. To improve your chances of staying as physically or mentally well as possible, there are a few things you can do, including the following:

Eat as healthily as you can

A balanced diet can help improve and maintain your physical health as well as your mental well-being and mood.

- At least five portions of a variety of fruit and veg every day to provide a range of vitamins, minerals and other valuable nutrients. If you fall short of this target regularly or just occasionally, you could consider taking a good quality multivitamin and mineral supplement that provides decent levels of important nutrients. There's even some evidence that taking a multivitamin could help boost your mood and improve your feelings of well-being .

- Starchy foods – preferably higher-fibre wholegrain varieties (potatoes with their skins on, wholewheat pasta and brown rice, for instance).

- Some dairy or dairy alternatives (ideally lower-fat varieties) to provide protein and calcium for healthy teeth and bones.

- Some non-dairy protein such as fish, poultry or lean meats, or plant-based sources of protein such as beans, peas and lentils. You should also aim to eat at least two portions of fish each week, one of which should be oily. If, however, you don't like eating fish you could try a high-strength fish oil supplement, as the omega-3 fatty acids found in oily fish such as salmon, trout, herring, mackerel and sardines have been linked with a range of physical and mental health benefits.

Vegetarian and vegan omega-3 supplements are also more widely available these days. These supplements source their active ingredients from plant organisms called microalgae rather than fish.

Oily fish are also one of the few foods that supply us with vitamin D, which we need for several important functions including better calcium absorption and healthy immunity. However many people in this country may not be getting enough vitamin D, especially during the winter months. That's why official UK guidelines recommend everyone consider taking a daily vitamin D supplement from October to March, with some people who have very little or no sun exposure or those with dark skin advised to take a supplement all year round (xvix).

If you want to take a vitamin D supplement the recommended form is vitamin D3 (cholecalciferol), as this is the natural form of vitamin D our bodies make when we're exposed to sunlight. You can get these in tablet form as well as in veggie-friendly drops. Most vitamin D3 supplements aren't suitable for vegans, however, since they're made from the fat of lamb's wool. But the good news is you can get vegan vitamin D3 supplements available these days that are sourced from lichen.

- Small amounts of fats, ideally mostly healthier unsaturated fats such as vegetable, rapeseed, olive and sunflower oils.

- Only occasional small amounts of foods high in sugar and fat, such as chocolate, biscuits, cakes, butter and ice cream.

Get plenty of exercise

This doesn't mean you have to join a gym or start training for a marathon. Just stay as active as you can – even a quick 10-minute stroll will help improve your energy levels and your mood. To support your physical and mental wellbeing, try to achieve the target of 150 minutes of moderate activity each week (or gradually work up to it if you need to). Achieving 150 minutes a week shouldn't be difficult – it can work out as little as three 10-minute bursts a day on five days of the week if you don't have time for more prolonged activities.

If you have a physical or mental health condition, check with your GP before you start, especially if you're taking any medication (some medicines can affect the type and amount of physical activity that's safe for you to do).

Also, remember: any exercise you do counts towards your target, even if it's just walking to the shops, dancing around your living room or tidying up your garden. Plus you don't have to do vigorous exercise – more gentle activities are also beneficial, such as yoga, t'ai chi or walking the dog.

Tackle your stress levels

Good nutrition and regular physical activity can also help you manage chronic stress and the effects it can have on your mind and body. Other things that could help you cope with stress more effectively include spending time outdoors in green spaces, practising mindfulness or meditation, having plenty of social interaction and getting lots of good-quality sleep (try reading our guide to sleep and insomnia for tips on sleeping better if you struggle to get a regular eight hours a night).

Give up smoking

According to the Mental Health Foundation, smoking has a negative impact on both mental and physical health (iv). Even if you smoke because you feel it helps you cope with stress or other mental health issues, the truth is the effects don't last, and smoking is likely to make you feel worse in the long run. If you're a smoker, quitting is also the best thing you can do for your physical health.

The good news is there's never been a better time to stop smoking, thanks to the variety of stop smoking aids available that are designed to help – by relieving nicotine withdrawal symptoms for instance (products are widely available and include nicotine patches, gum and lozenges).

Mental Health Myths and Facts

Can you tell the difference between a mental health myth and fact? Learn more about the most common mental health myths and information to help de-stigmatize them. **SAMHSA** works to prevent and treat mental health conditions and provides support for people seeking or already in recovery.

Myth: Mental health issues can't affect me.

Fact: Mental health issues can affect anyone. In 2020, about:

- One in 5 American adults experienced a mental health condition in a given year
- One in 6 young people have experienced a major depressive episode
- One in 20 Americans have lived with a serious mental illness, such as schizophrenia, bipolar disorder, or major depression

Additionally, suicide is a leading cause of death in the United States. In fact, it was the second leading cause of death for people ages 10-24. Suicide has accounted for the loss of more than 45,979 American lives in 2020, nearly double the number of lives lost to homicide.

Myth: Children don't experience mental health issues.

Myth: People with mental health conditions are violent.

Myth: People with mental health needs, even those who are managing their mental health conditions, cannot tolerate the stress of holding down a job.

Myth: Mental health issues are a result of personality weakness or character flaws, and people can "snap out of it" if they try hard enough.

Myth: There is no hope for people with mental health issues. Once a friend or family member develops a mental health condition, they will never recover.

Myth: Therapy and self-help are a waste of time. Why bother when you can just take a pill?

Myth: I can't do anything for a person with a mental health issue.

Myth: It is impossible to prevent a mental health condition.

Physical activity: the way ahead for a healthier India - Ammar Suhail

To the Editor,

Physical inactivity is a global health problem with considerable healthcare and economic burden. Various studies show a strong association between physical inactivity and the development of **non-communicable diseases (NCDs)** . Physical inactivity has a negative effect on mental health and quality of life as well. Globally, the NCDs have replaced **communicable diseases (CDs)** as a cause for mortality. NCD-related deaths have increased exponentially; WHO estimates that over 80% of them occur in low- and middle-income countries (LMICs). The published literature to date suggests an epidemic of physical inactivity and NCDs in India. India is almost contributing two thirds of the mortality due to NCDs in the South-East Asia Region. The additional worrying fact is that NCDs are developing a decade earlier in the Indian population than individuals in the developed nations. There are multifactorial reasons for such a rise, though physical inactivity is considered the most crucial factor for this NCDs epidemic .

Indeed, this global burden of NCDs is caused due to physical inactivity, and we suggest that focus on physical activity (PA) is the way ahead. We must discuss in what ways we can move forward and promote PA to impact the public health.

The way ahead

PA has already been proven to help prevent and manage different NCDs . PA has also shown evidence in the reduction of NCDs associated with premature deaths . The best way forward is to promote PA at a population level. According to the literature, PA is emphasized as the most robust intervention to decrease risks associated with NCDs' development. Despite the fact, there is a decrease in the number of physically active individuals. The **Indian Council of Medical Research–India Diabetes (ICMR–INDIAB)** study reports a large percentage of people in India are inactive, with fewer than 10% engaging in recreational physical activity . The increasing economic development, improvement in transportation methods, and other technological advancements further increase the level of physical inactivity .

The NCD interventions can be addressed at two levels: population-based interventions and individual-based interventions. Population-based interventions focus on reducing NCD risk factors, and individual-based interventions focus on NCDs in primary care settings . The integration of both approaches is needed to tackle the widespread increase of NCDs . Improving physical activity at the population level may bring a 6 to 10% downfall in major NCDs . In the Indian context, the lack of people participating in physical activity can be attributed to various reasons. The way forward should be addressing all these reasons to achieve the desired levels of PA. National health portal in response to the new **Global Action Plan on Physical Activity (GAPPA)** 2018–2030 suggest reductions in physical inactivity by 25% by 2025 .

Increasing physical activity requires a systems-based approach—it cannot be a single policy solution . In a country like India which has the greatest diversity, this must be done at various levels. The increased level of PA in a society can be achieved through three methods; one of them should be promoting PA at the national level, aided by a national policy targeted at such interventions. There is a need to formulate a national physical activity program to appropriately promote physical activity at the population level so that lacunae could be bridged . Secondly, by incorporating PA and its benefits in our education system, to imbibe PA in the social and cultural norms of the society. A recent study proposed incorporating NCD risk reduction strategies and practical sessions on health promotion and behavior change activities in the health professional education system. The research also suggests that our curriculum lacks focus on healthcare promotion and long-term physical activity .

Thirdly, there is a need to understand our environments, as they will play a role in facilitating PA . WHO suggests that creating active environments must achieve a 15% reduction in physical inactivity by 2025. This reduction is a crucial step to curb the rise of NCDs. The strategy of building physical activity facilitating environments will replicate in terms of active people and active societies. Better environments can be created by strengthening road safety, improving access to public open spaces, improving walking and cycling networks, and implementing proactive building policies . These strategies of building physical activity enabling environments will replicate in terms of active people and active societies.

The other factors that need to be addressed are barriers, beliefs, and myths associated with PA and NCDs to ensure better PA participation. The studies exploring PA barriers in the Indian context highlight social and cultural norms such as females face social censuring for participating in PA . The majority of people believe that routine household activities are the same as PA . These beliefs and myths must be addressed at the community level. The barriers differ among age groups, and this should be considered while designing policies for different age groups. In adolescence, physical inactivity is associated with electronic gadgets and lethargy, while in middle-aged females, it is related to lack of time, motivation, and interest . Considering this system-based approach of addressing all the factors is the right way ahead. PA can be used as a preventive tool to curb the epidemic rise of NCDs.

In every health care system, preventive measures reduce chances of further damage, improve quality of life, and yet remain cost-effective. Physical activity can be deemed an easy, efficient, and most affordable method for the population.

How much physical activity do adults need?

Physical activity is anything that gets your body moving. Each week adults need 150 minutes of moderate-intensity physical activity and 2 days of muscle strengthening activity, according to the current **Physical Activity Guidelines.**

Some Activity is Better than None

We know 150 minutes of physical activity each week sounds like a lot, but you don't have to do it all at once. It could be 30 minutes a day, 5 days a week. You can spread your activity out during the week and break it up into smaller chunks of time.

Stay active: It can make life better.

Physical activity supports physical and mental health. The benefits of physical activity make it one of the most important things you can do for your health.

Move more and Sit less

Adults should move more and sit less throughout the day. Some physical activity is better than none. Adults who sit less and do any amount of moderate-to-vigorous intensity physical activity gain some health benefits.

What health risks are linked to physical inactivity?

Lack of physical activity has clearly been shown to be a risk factor for cardiovascular disease and other conditions:

- Less active and less fit people have a greater risk of developing high blood pressure.

- Physical activity can reduce your risk for type 2 diabetes.

- Studies show that physically active people are less likely to develop coronary heart disease than those who are inactive. This is even after researchers accounted for smoking, alcohol use, and diet.

- Lack of physical activity can add to feelings of anxiety and depression.

- Physical inactivity may increase the risk of certain cancers.

- Physically active overweight or obese people significantly reduced their risk for disease with regular physical activity.

- Older adults who are physically active can reduce their risk for falls and improve their ability to do daily activities.

Facts about inactive lifestyles

Thousands and thousands of deaths occur each year due to a lack of regular physical activity. In addition:

- Inactivity tends to increase with age.

- Women are more likely to lead inactive lifestyles than men.

- Non-Hispanic white adults are more likely to engage in physical activity than Hispanic and black adults.

*****